Experiencing Acupuncture

by the same author

The Spirit of the Organs
Twelve stories for practitioners and patients
ISBN 978 1 84819 378 9
eISBN 978 0 85701 334 7

Intuitive Acupuncture
ISBN 978 1 84819 273 7
eISBN 978 0 85701 220 3

Acupuncture for New Practitioners
ISBN 978 1 84819 102 0
eISBN 978 0 85701 083 4

Zero Balancing
Touching the Energy of Bone
Foreword by Fritz Smith, MD FCC Ac
Illustrated by Gina Michaels
ISBN 978 1 84819 234 8
eISBN 978 0 85701 182 4

of related interest

Acupuncture Strategies for Complex Patients
From Consultation to Treatment
Skya Abbate, DOM
ISBN 978 1 84819 380 2
eISBN 978 0 85701 336 1

Experiencing Acupuncture

Journeys of Body, Mind and Spirit for Patients and Practitioners

John Hamwee

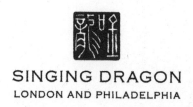

SINGING DRAGON

LONDON AND PHILADELPHIA

Every effort has been made to trace copyright holders and to obtain
their permission for the use of copyright material where necessary to
do so. The author and the publisher apologize for any omissions and
would be grateful if notified of any acknowledgements that should
be incorporated in future reprints or editions of this book.

First published in 2020
by Singing Dragon
an imprint of Jessica Kingsley Publishers
73 Collier Street
London N1 9BE, UK
and
400 Market Street, Suite 400
Philadelphia, PA 19106, USA

www.singingdragon.com

Copyright © John Hamwee 2020
Painting on cover © Jennie Foley 2002

Library of Congress Cataloging in Publication Data
A CIP catalog record for this book is available from the Library of Congress

British Library Cataloguing in Publication Data
A CIP catalogue record for this book is available from the British Library

ISBN 978 1 78775 250 4
eISBN 978 1 78775 251 1

Printed and bound in Great Britain

For Dorsett

Acknowledgements

Kathryn Cave, Myra Connell, Polly McAfee, Sophie Mitchell, Cathy Nicholson and James Unsworth all took time and trouble to comment on early drafts of the book and made many valuable comments and suggestions. Readers will be grateful to them as I am. Darren Harris and Natasa Bertalanic gave generously of their special knowledge.

Jessica Kingsley has been the best publisher any author could wish for, and I thank her for all the support and encouragement she has given me over many years. And I thank James Cherry at Singing Dragon for receiving the book with enthusiasm and championing it with great persistence.

I am glad to have this opportunity to acknowledge once again the debt I owe to my teachers – Meriel Darby, Angie Hicks and Dr Fritz Smith. I draw endlessly on their wisdom as I work and write.

And I owe the inspiration for this book, as for most of the others I have written, to Dorsett Edmunds, master practitioner and true friend.

Contents

Note to Readers

All the accounts of treatment in this book come directly from my experience in the treatment room. I have had to protect the privacy of my patients and the confidentiality of our work together, so I have concealed their identities in various ways – changing gender, age and background details and sometimes conflating the experiences of two or three of them into one story. In two instances, where full concealment was not possible, the patients read the accounts and gave consent to them being published. But everything I report really did happen, and all the stories are true.

The accounts are grouped into three sets of three, as there are common themes in the experience of treating the patients in each group, but the accounts can be read in any order. And there is no technical information in the book which would come as a surprise to someone who has ever had acupuncture, and very little which would be puzzling to any other reader. Practitioners, however, may be interested in some more technical detail and so the appendix gives a brief account of my reasons for doing specific treatments and the points I used in them.

Introduction

The Experience of Treatment

Two experiences of treatment opened my eyes to a new way of seeing the world. One was as a patient. The first time I had acupuncture was for some minor ailment. It improved, but what astonished me was that my life-long asthma disappeared. My acupuncturist seemed unsurprised: 'If you get better then everything will get better,' she commented. It struck me then as simple common sense, but at the same time it was profoundly radical for it was the opposite of everything I had been told about illness – and I had been ill a lot as a child.

The other experience was soon after I had qualified as an acupuncturist and zero balancer. A woman told me that she had broken her left arm in a car crash two years earlier. According to the X rays the fracture had healed perfectly and her doctors could find no evidence of nerve damage, and yet she could hardly use her left hand. It moved as directed by her brain, if a little slowly, but it was not strong enough to allow her to pick up a cup or to drive a car. I felt along the arm and it was remarkable. Above the site of the fracture it felt warm and alive, but below it was cold and dead.

Fortunately I had been taught by Dr Fritz Smith, a master practitioner with an unusual set of qualifications, for he is a

Western medical doctor, osteopath and acupuncturist. Before I met him I already knew that there are coherent and organised flows of energy in the body, flows which were mapped thousands of years ago and which have been used by practitioners in the East ever since; what I didn't know was that with a little practice it is possible to feel these flows and to sense if they have been disturbed or interrupted. I could tell that the flow down this woman's arm had been broken along with the bone, so her hand was not receiving the energy it needed to work properly. Could I re-establish that flow?

I had never done it before but, relying on the methods Dr Smith had taught me, it turned out to be easy, and within a few minutes her hand started to re-gain its strength. I was more surprised than the patient. It is one thing to know the theory; it is another to see it work so quickly and conclusively.

These two experiences showed me the enormous scope of a system of medicine which seeks to heal through changing the state of a patient's energy. One treatment was for the chronic weakness of an organ, the other for a failure of a limb; one condition was not specifically treated at all, while the other was treated very locally and deliberately; one kind of treatment I could learn from the ancient texts, the other only from a master. But what they all had in common is that they showed me that if the energy of the body is restored to at least something approaching its natural flows, its rhythms and vitality, then healing is possible.

They also stimulated in me an interest in the experience of treatment. Books about acupuncture usually set out the theory and explain the concepts used in diagnosis, while some also describe various techniques as well. This book is completely different. It tries to capture what acupuncture is like. It does so through accounts of the treatment of a few of my patients – stories of the journeys they undertook in order to get well. Remarkable, sometimes inspiring stories of healing; stories too of the doubts and difficulties I often had in treating them; and stories of failures as well.

I hope that these accounts will help those who are considering treatment for the first time and want to know what they might be letting themselves in for. And those who are already having acupuncture may have wondered, as one of my patients once wondered out loud: 'What are you doing as you think about how to treat me? Are you evaluating me in some way, judging me, trying to work out the cause of my illness? Does it matter that we get on well? And why do you write so many notes?' The accounts should also help patients to make the most of their treatments. They show that, contrary to popular belief, acupuncture has much more to offer than pain relief or an improvement in symptoms, and they make it clear that healing often comes about through a particular kind of collaboration between patient and practitioner.

I hope that these accounts have something to offer to acupuncturists as well. I often think how much I would like to be a fly on the wall of someone else's treatment room and see how he or she works with a patient who, for example, comes with an enormous list of symptoms, or who only gives the briefest of answers to questions, or who doesn't respond well to treatment in spite of a convincing diagnosis and treatment strategy – all common experiences for me. I hope that my frank accounts of how I tried to work with the uncertainties and anxieties we all face may help other acupuncturists cope with their own.

So the book gives nine full accounts of acupuncture treatments, each one showing what the experience was like as a patient and I travelled together along the sometimes rocky road towards health. A few of the patients had physical pain or dysfunction; some had mental or emotional pain too; and treatment for others was really about reviving their spirit. The journey was different each time, for as a consultant neurologist points out, 'Everybody's experience of illness is their own...

A person's personality and their life experience moulds the clinical presentation, the response and the outcome of any brush with illness' (O'Sullivan 2015, p.21). And the author might have added another thing which 'moulds the outcome' – the singular nature of the relationship between the patient and practitioner.

All of which raises a really interesting issue because medical education and textbooks, whether Western or Eastern, depend on generalisations; that is, on classifying types of illnesses and then types of treatments appropriate to each. There are the signs and symptoms of asthma or Crohn's disease, for example, in Western medicine and of Liver Qi Stagnation or Blood deficiency in Eastern, and they apply regardless of the individual differences of individual patients. So how to bridge the gap between these necessary generalisations and the equally necessary unique responses to the particular patient?

One answer is for experienced practitioners to report on what they actually do and how they try to bridge that gap.

> The focus of the case study is on understanding what happens for the individual, following his or her story, seeking patterns and connections, and drawing out meanings…analyses of case histories provide deep insights not into medicine as a system but into medicine as it is actually practised, with all its diversity, subtle nuances, unexplained happenings, varied interpretations and wealth of potential meanings. (MacPherson 1997, pp.6–7)

In the accounts of acupuncture treatments which make up the bulk of the book there is plenty of the diversity referred to in this quotation. Some lasted a few weeks while others went on for years; there are unlikely successes and unexpected disappointments; there are common conditions and strange symptoms; there are patients who worked hard to get well and those who chose not to participate in trying to recover their health.

There are plenty of unexplained happenings too, as I struggled to understand my patients' responses not only to my treatments but also to my questions, explanations and suggestions. And finally there is a wealth of potential meanings in these accounts, for as well as the meanings which occurred to me and my patients there will be more that occur to you as you notice things I did not see, as you compare my experiences with your own, whether as patient or practitioner, and as you mull over what happened to each of these people in their journeys towards health.

When patients ask the perfectly reasonable question – How does acupuncture work? – there is no one simple answer. Partly it has to do with the flows of energy in the body and with the accurate diagnosis of their disturbance – topics covered in all the textbooks. But partly it also has to do with experiences which are rarely described or discussed. For example, it makes the most enormous difference if the patient really commits to treatment and is willing to change old habits which would undermine any healing. So how does a practitioner stimulate that commitment and motivate the patient to overcome those habits? Then there are patients whose illness appears to be psychosomatic, at least in part, or who make themselves ill through worrying about their every symptom however small or temporary; how to help them overcome the unconscious barrier to health?

There seems to be no better way to learn how to do these kinds of things than to read accounts of how an experienced practitioner tackled them:

> the clinical story is intended to improve clinical judgment…an intellectual virtue that depends not only on knowledge and skill but also on an innate thoughtfulness and decision-making ability … Neither medicine nor information science has improved on the story as a means of ordering and storing the experience of human and medical complexity. (Hunter 1986, p.619)

The great thing about true stories is that there is bound to be more in them than the writer ever imagined or intended. And they are bound to strike different readers differently too, as they will each take from them what has meaning and value for them in their own lives. Reading stories like the ones that follow is, then, a fine way to appreciate the unique experience of acupuncture.

1

William's Irritable Bowel and Getting Energy to Flow

WILLIAM WAS A SURPRISE. HE CAN'T HAVE BEEN more than nineteen or twenty, and he was huge. A tree trunk of a man, well over six feet tall and wide with it. Yet there was no sense of power in him. Instead he looked a little timid, abashed, as if he'd been caught out being too big or too strong and wanted to apologise for it. He'd booked by email, so I didn't know what I was expecting, but it wasn't this.

I waited for him on the front step of the porch, thinking that he was going to have to practically crawl to get through the front door and along the corridor to my treatment room. Old Westmoreland farmhouses were not built for the likes of him.

I always stand there, waiting for patients to park, ready to greet them as they get out of the car, lock it, and walk towards me. Why do I do this? Why not wait inside until they knock on the door? The same goes for offering patients a drink when they arrive, which I always do. Why do I do many of the things that make up my normal working day? I don't really know. They are habits, a kind of style.

I'm not sure if these things make a difference, and I ought to have some idea because once a week I also work in a doctor's surgery in London where I can't stand by the door and welcome people in, nor can I offer them a drink, let alone make them a cup of tea. So it should be easy to compare the two. But that's central London, and home is in a hamlet in the Lake District surrounded by fields and sheep; there are so many variables that who can say what difference anything makes? And that's just the very first moments. The same holds true for all that follows.

I'm old enough to be William's grandfather – what effect does that have? The thought returns when I find out that he was very close to his grandfather and misses him dreadfully since the old man died. Will that help William to trust me and to respond well to the treatment? And then there is my invariable uniform – smart navy trousers and a white shirt. Would it be better if I wore a white coat? I know some patients would prefer it but it is a bit too medical for my taste.

William sits down opposite me and looks at his hands. I sense a weariness in him for this is a story he has told many times to many people and none of them have made a difference. So it occurs to me that the usual kind of bland questions with which I often start – How can I help? or What are your symptoms like? – won't awaken his enthusiasm for treatment; instead I say that I am going to carry out some diagnostic tests, like looking at his tongue and taking his pulses. I feel a slight quickening of his interest when, after seeing his tongue twice, I turn away from him to make a few notes. Unusually I also take his pulses with him still sitting in his chair. I don't want him on the couch just yet – we still need to talk and I don't want to do that with him lying down looking up at me. As I move away to make notes again he glances at me, the first time he has risked meeting my eye. I suppose that, for him, at least all this is new.

I already have a wealth of information. His tongue is a good shape but it is pale, and at the back there is a distinctly sticky yellowish film – all is not well in his intestines. And his pulses are a shock for they are the pulses of a different man, an older, weaker man, one depleted by illness or over-work. I try pressing down on the pulses to see if there is any inner strength or resilience but I am simply squashing them to nothing. I feel sympathy and concern for this young man. At his age he should be relishing life to the full but it is quite clear that he simply isn't able to.

'You must get very tired,' I say. He looks at me again. He is suspicious – is this a trick? – but he likes the sympathy. Suddenly a word comes to me – truculent. For some reason it seems to fit.

This happens quite often with a patient. A word arrives unbidden and feels right, as if no other word would convey the vague and formless impression I have of the person in front of me. Although I treat these quick insights with caution as they are not always true, I often find them helpful. With this young man, the word does crystallise something about the contrast between his size and his way of being, and it does show me that I may need to lead him along slowly.

'How long has this been going on?' I ask.

'Three years, nearly four.'

I am shocked. In his late teenage years, when he needed to be doing A levels, playing sport, travelling, meeting girls, having fun, he has been unwell. What effect has it had on him? Does he get depressed? Has he become solitary?

'What's the most difficult thing about it?' I continue, even though I don't yet know what the 'it' is.

He considers. This is a person who takes any question seriously and gives it due deliberation. He is taking his time; trying to choose. Finally he says, 'I have to miss lectures and then I've got to catch up afterwards.'

'Because...?'

'I have to go to the toilet and it's urgent.'

'You have to go more than once an hour?' I can't keep surprise out of my voice.

'Can be three or four times an hour. I can't keep walking in and out of lectures.'

I start to imagine the effect this must have on the life of a young man. 'So you can't go to the cinema either?'

'No, I do. It's normally much better in the evening. And I sit on the end of a row.'

'You go with friends, or a girlfriend?'

'Usually with Rachel, my girlfriend. She doesn't mind. She's used to it.'

'Have you been together long?'

Although he gives a straightforward answer, 'Two years, come September', he looks a bit puzzled. What has this to do with his bowels?

I don't want to startle him, so I decide to go down more familiar lines. I ask him what he is taking for his condition. Another shock. As well as the pretty obvious, and as far as I know harmless, remedies, like Imodium and Psyllium, he is also on Amitriptyline, a strong anti-depressant. Was this prescribed, I wonder, because he has been depressed or because one of its common side effects is constipation?

'Do they help?'

'Not really. No.'

I need to pause. I think he is feeling slightly pressurised, so asking more questions isn't going to relax him enough to give me fuller answers. Instead I decide to take his pulses again. For one thing, it provides me with something to do while I absorb what I have learnt to far, and it gives a bit of quiet time for my intuition to come up with something helpful. And the pulses often change after ten minutes or so and start to show more of the true picture.

I find that his pulses are indeed a little fuller than before, so he is not quite as depleted as I first thought. But now that the others have lifted a bit, it is all the more obvious that his heart and small intestine pulses are really low. I check his spleen pulse again; because the spleen channel feeds into the heart channel it may be that there is some kind of blockage between them and energy isn't reaching his heart as it should. And indeed there is a tight quality to the spleen pulse, as if energy is dammed up in the channel. I wonder what caused this blockage and I wonder too if his bowel trouble might start a bit higher up the digestive process, in the small intestine rather than the large.

What to do next? I certainly don't have a diagnosis yet, and I would like to learn a lot more about his emotional life before I start to treat him. On the other hand, perhaps I have enough information to make a start and to do something that will help; and that might give him the confidence to open up to me. After all, I can't expect a young man to come into the treatment room of a perfect stranger and within fifteen minutes start talking about deep fears and anxieties, let alone a past trauma.

I decide to ask him if he played sport at school. He looks like a sportsman and anyway I hope that I might learn more from his response to any topic other than his bowel. For the more time I spend in his presence the more I sense that he is carrying the burden of some deep unease or consuming worry.

At the mention of sport there is an immediate change in him. Now he is confident, now he sits up straighter, now he meets my eye and, for the first time, words flow out of him. It was rowing. He was so good at it that he was given a scholarship to a prestigious public school and he rowed for Great Britain in the junior world championship where he won a gold medal. He was captain of the crew when they travelled to events in Asia, South Africa and America, and in spite of difficult conditions and technical problems with the boat – which he explained at some length – they won every regatta they entered. I ask him what kind of boat he rowed in and what position he occupied in the boat. Again, he is eloquent. This is his passion.

I am delighted. Here is a part of him I need to get to know and it is an important corrective to my first impression of a downtrodden man. Actually not quite a man, for in spite of his size there is still something boyish about him. And it occurs to me that he has only mentioned being in the junior championships when surely at his age he would now be in the senior ones. How to approach this? I am not quite sure. Meanwhile there is one obvious question.

'How do you manage in a boat when you need to go to the toilet all the time?'

'It's difficult.'

I wait. There is clearly more to say, so I wait for him to say it. Then what comes is unexpected.

'It was in Hong Kong. The final. I was alright in the heats. But as we were about to get into the boat to paddle down to the start I knew I had to go to the toilet. I told the coach. He said there wasn't time. It made me angry and I swore at him. He took me out of the boat and put the reserve in. I came home early. I never rowed again, not properly.'

I was shocked. One moment, and his career came crashing down. Now he can no longer do the sport he loved and at which he excelled. That is hard. It must have broken his heart and I can imagine that life has been a struggle ever since. Though, I reflect, it doesn't answer the question which lies at the back of my mind – what set all this off in the first place? Whatever it was, perhaps that was the real heartbreaker? And the truculence I noticed earlier – did it arise through resentment and disappointment at what happened in Hong Kong, or was it there before? Maybe the coach reacted as he did because William had been truculent with him.

Then I remind myself that my job is not to help William understand his psychological state and that, at least for now, I must resist the temptation to go further down this road. My job is to get to know how his energy works when he is well, and how it has stopped working now he is unwell.

I look at him afresh and ask myself, 'What is his energy like?' And immediately I know that it is delicate, fragile, sensitive. It comes to me in a flash, but it is the conclusion my mind has drawn from a hundred different fragments of information: the weakness of his pulses, the way he shrinks into himself, my instinct to tread very carefully with my questions, and so on. And it is crucial knowledge. Given his size and strength, it would be easy to assume that his energy is robust and treat him accordingly, and I am sure that nothing would happen if I did. On the contrary, it has to be coaxed towards change, has to be persuaded that feeling more comfortable is a possibility, and needs to be encouraged to flow freely and easily. If it was forced or bludgeoned or pushed about, it would simply retreat into its shell and become unavailable to me and my needles.

And, as so often, I realise that completely unconsciously I have hit upon an image which is helpful. The phrase 'retreating into his shell' conjures up a picture of a crab pulling its claws underneath its hard carapace. There is indeed a hard shell to William but that is because he feels so vulnerable inside. I am starting to understand why his bowel is over-sensitive; it is because he is.

Which makes me think of another patient I have treated. At first sight the two of them couldn't be more different. Rich is outgoing, charming, confident. He spent his thirties doing something complicated in finance and by the time he was in his early forties he was extremely wealthy and had appalling trouble with his bowel. It was so bad he had to give up work altogether and could barely walk a hundred yards. I asked him what the worst thing was about his condition and he told me that he was too ill to play with his children.

What Rich and William had in common is that they had both been subject to long-term pressure. At work, Rich could gain or lose millions in minutes, and so could the people who worked under him and for whom he was responsible. Every day, he was on a knife edge between success and failure. As for William, so much was expected of him and at such a young age – the school scholarship, the endless round of training and championships, the demands of being captain of the crew – that as a consequence his energy had become depleted. Both of them had driven themselves so hard that they had used up all their reserves and they had got to the point where their systems could not cope with the slightest extra strain. Any addition to the load and, like the last straw on the camel's back, something would crack.

Which leaves the intriguing question, why did their systems fail in this particular way – why an irritable bowel rather than, say, asthma or a stomach ulcer?

There are two kinds of answers to that question, one specific and one general. First, the general. We all have typical illnesses; we all crack somewhere. Sometimes it is possible to trace it back to a childhood trauma of some kind; I have a patient with chronic stomach problems which I am pretty sure started when he was put on solids at three weeks old – a crazy demand to put on a baby's digestion. Or a child may be brought up in a damp house with parents who smoke, leaving the lungs vulnerable for the rest of his or her life. Or there may be some genetic weakness. Perhaps one of these was true for both William and Rich.

There is a more specific reason too. The bowel works best with order and regularity. That is why it tends to go awry after long-haul flights which cross time zones. It has to be able to hold onto the faeces for quite a long time until they are properly formed and then, in an abrupt reversal of energy, be able to let them go quickly. It isn't hard to imagine that this process is controlled by some kind of inner clock; keep changing the time when it expects to let go and it gets confused.

To most Western doctors this would seem a peculiar explanation. For them, dysfunctions of the kind that William and

Rich suffer from arise either from germs or viruses. Germs would seem the more likely cause, and indeed both men were prescribed antibiotics – in Rich's case in ever increasing amounts until, by the time I first saw him, he was taking well over the normal limit. His doctor's theory seemed to be that if it wasn't working it must be because he wasn't taking enough to overcome the bacteria – so he had to keep taking more. There is a problem with this theory, or rather two problems. One is that there is no logical place to stop upping the dose – at what point does the doctor admit that the diagnosis is wrong? And the other problem is that antibiotics at that level, and taken for that amount of time, do a lot of damage. If they are saving life, as they do, then the side effects are irrelevant; but in Rich's case they were compounding his problems.

We humans are good at prioritising. If a child is in danger, for example, we forget everything and race to the rescue, and there are many accounts of people suddenly acquiring superhuman strength when they need to free a person trapped by fallen debris. Our minds focus on the one task and our bodies ignore all other demands in order to complete it. That is also the case for athletes who have to be at the top of their mental and physical powers, ready to go at whatever time has been fixed for their event. And the same is true for a city trader who has to respond in the moment to sudden fluctuations in the market – everything else is put aside and ignored. Consequently, when the body is required to perform again at a time of the athlete's or the trader's choosing, it can't necessarily respond on demand, nor respond sufficiently quickly before the next event or the next flurry of activity which requires full attention. In these circumstances it isn't hard to see how an organ which thrives on regularity and consistency can lose its ability to function normally.

So there I am, sitting opposite William, and thinking that while I am far from having a full diagnosis of his condition I do know enough to do a treatment which will start to help him.

Now I have to choose between what the Chinese call a root treatment or a branch treatment. The first goes to the fundamental cause of the condition. It tends to take time to produce a change in the patient's symptoms but in the long run is the route to lasting change. The branch treatment, on the other hand, is designed largely to relieve the patient's symptoms. It has its advantages. For one thing it is what the patient has come for; and for another the patient is more likely to trust the practitioner and to trust acupuncture when there are some quick results, and so keep coming long enough to have the root treatments too.

It may seem obvious that the best course of action is to do some branch treatments first to win the patient's confidence, and then go on to the deeper level. It is obvious really, but experienced practitioners know that there are times when, for reasons we may not fully understand, we are drawn to do the opposite. This was one of those times. With lots of ideas buzzing around in my head which I don't have time to assemble into any coherent order, and acutely aware that nearly half of the hour of his appointment has gone and I haven't started to needle him – and there is another patient coming straight after, there isn't time to think it all out. I have to trust my instinct.

And my instinct tells me that the blockage in the flow of energy between his spleen and his heart is fundamental, and that nothing will change until it is removed. So I choose to needle acupuncture points which will re-establish the normal circulation of energy from the spleen to the heart. This has nothing directly to do with his bowel, so it definitely counts as a root treatment.

As I get out my needles I think again that his symptom might really be coming from distress in the small intestine rather than the large. For one thing, the small intestine is the organ which carries out almost all of the absorption of nourishment into the body; and for another the health and illness of the heart and small intestine are very closely linked in Chinese medicine.

Perhaps there is some connection between the small intestine struggling to cope and the heart feeling starved of the emotional nourishment it needs.

It is all starting to make sense. Again, it isn't really a diagnosis but it is a hypothesis. The test of that hypothesis will be the treatment itself – will he respond positively or will it have no noticeable effect?

I show him the needles and tell him where I am going to put them. He looks a little bemused, which is understandable, as the first point is high on the side of his torso and the second is in his armpit, a weird enough place in any event and more than a little difficult to relate to his bowel symptoms. As I bend down to find the exact location of the point I catch an odour coming off him. I can't quite identify it – it might be sweet or burning or some combination. It would be useful diagnostic information, but in the moment I can't put a label to it; perhaps it will come to me later.

The needles slip in easily, which makes me think I have hit the points alright. But still, there is always that slight anxiety, especially the first time. How will he react? Is this what he needs? Might it aggravate his condition? I almost hold my breath waiting to find out.

Usually, I only get an answer to these questions when I take the patient's pulses again and see how they have responded; and sometimes I have to wait until the next session for feedback – but not with William. Within moments of the needles going in he starts to laugh – though the word is too flat and dull for what he is doing. It is a rumbling, gurgling merriment, welling up from deep inside him, and it bursts out like lava from a volcano. He apologises. He is embarrassed but he is grinning. Whatever it is, it is irresistibly funny. In any case there is nothing he can do about it because it is completely involuntary and utterly uncontrollable. It dies down for a moment or two, then breaks out again. Now there are tears as well as the laughter.

This goes on for what seems like a long time, but when I look at my watch I see that it hasn't lasted much more than five minutes. I check his pulses again and I am delighted to feel that the spleen pulse has now softened and no longer has that pushy quality which spoke of a blockage. The heart pulse has responded as I hoped and is now almost as strong as the others. What's more, I am pleased to see that all the other pulses have improved, which tells me that once the blockage has been removed there is nothing else stopping the free and proper flow of energy round his body.

His laughter is such a strong involuntary response to the needles that it has to signify at least the start of change; and not some irrelevant change either, for the laughter expresses joy and relief. So I am as sure as I can be that William will get better, though I don't know how long it will take.

This was a turning point for me as an acupuncturist. Previously, I had seen all sorts of responses to the needles but never anything remotely like this uncontrollable, infectious laughter. Unarguably, the needles had caused it, and caused it instantly too. And unarguably his response told me that it was good for him. So the completely reasonable doubts I had as a relatively new practitioner – can hair-thin needles in a couple of points, for example, really make such a difference? – were dispelled in an instant.

Very early in my training I had been taught the fundamental idea that lies behind all forms of acupuncture – that health is when someone's energy is flowing freely and naturally. And even if a person does fall ill, for sometimes the body's defences are overwhelmed by pathogens, recovery will be quicker and easier if energy is flowing properly. I also knew the theory behind removing blocks such as the one between the spleen and heart channels. But there is all the difference in the world between learning an idea passed down through generations of practitioners and expounded in the textbooks, and seeing it happening under your own hands in your own treatment room. From the moment William's laughter subsided I knew that if I could only find out how to restore the proper circulation of their energy, most of my patients would get better.

William looks bemused as he gets up from the couch and sits down opposite me again. He shakes his head. He doesn't know what has happened, but whatever it was it was really strange. He doesn't know if it is good or bad, helpful or irrelevant, normal with acupuncture or unusual, or even some kind of trick. He looks at me with the remains of the huge smile that cracked his face when he was laughing and asks, 'What was that all about?'

It is a perfectly fair question but I don't know how to answer it. I can't tell him what I really think because in my head it comes as shorthand technical phrases which would make no sense to him at all. A full answer would take too long, even here, but the gist of it is as follows.

When there is an abrupt and profound change in a person's energy – which happens rarely – then the whole mind, body and spirit is jumped suddenly into a completely new state. And the shock of it is a bit like the shock of a really good joke. With most jokes, the first few sentences set up an expectation of what is going to come next. Then, suddenly and with a few brief words, that expectation is shown to be completely and utterly wrong and in that moment we realise that we have been going down the wrong track all along. We also see that the conclusion of the joke is, at one and the same time, both completely unexpected and utterly obvious. Our involuntary response to the surprise of it all is to laugh.

So William has had a similar experience. He experienced his energy being suddenly jumped out of its old state and into a new and different one, and the surprise of it has made him laugh. What is more, he recognises, unconsciously and instinctively, that the new state is better than the old, so as well as the laughter there are tears of relief.

It is a complicated idea. It has taken me quite a long time to find a way of writing it clearly here and I am sure I wouldn't have been able to come up with nearly as good an explanation on the spur of the moment in the treatment room. And anyway, it isn't an explanation which would be helpful to him, especially as he is still recovering from the impact of the dramatic change in his energy. This is an example of a common enough dilemma – how to answer a question in a way which is both truthful and helpful, when a helpful answer may not be quite true and a truthful answer may not help.

I can't remember exactly what I said but it was something like 'It must seem ludicrous to you that after all this time, and after trying every kind of treatment and remedy, the answer should be a couple of hair-thin needles in your armpits – so ludicrous that it's funny.' Looking at this answer now, it seems to me to just about pass the test of being both sufficiently truthful (it does say something about the shock of it) and quite helpful (it suggests that even though the treatment is completely implausible it may still be the way back to health).

I can see William starting to think about my answer, for he is someone who feels the need to be conscientious and thorough about things – but to my relief I also see him give up. It won't serve him just yet to try to arrive at an understanding which will satisfy his rational mind; far better that for now he simply accepts what has happened to him and allows himself to adjust to it.

I then say the usual things I say to a patient after his or her first treatment. The need to notice any changes, not just changes in symptoms, so I can refine my diagnosis the next time. That people don't get better at a uniform rate, so it isn't sensible to get elated at immediate improvements nor downhearted if they are not sustained, the real test being whether there are fewer bad days, and they are less bad, and the good days are more frequent and better. He listens carefully, then we make another appointment.

I go ahead of him down the hallway, pointing out the places where he has to duck especially low. By the time he is standing on the limestone slab in front of the porch, towering over me, he has successfully avoided all five of them. Suddenly he says, 'Thank you', then reaches out his hand and shakes mine. For the first time there is trust in his eyes. I am pleased as I close the front door and go back to tidy my treatment room, for I feel we have made a start on creating a good relationship. There is no objective recipe for this, but there are two key ingredients which have to be in the mix. I felt completely committed to him and he had begun to trust me. For all the universality of the theories and techniques of acupuncture, for all the remarkable truth that the points do what the ancient books say they do, and just as accurately with an oarsman in Cumbria in the early twenty-first century as for a court official in China over a thousand years ago, still there is no doubt at all that the quality of the relationship between patient and practitioner makes the most enormous difference to the prospects of a successful outcome.

William got better. It took about five months of treatment, and there were certainly ups and downs along the way. From time to time, when under stress, his condition would return, though in a more manageable form, but most of the time he was fine. The last time I saw him he looked different. Gone was that boyish, bashful air that he used to carry about with him. He stood straighter, walked without his former shambling gait and had an air of confidence about him. It wasn't surprising, given that he was no longer the slave to a debilitating condition, but still it was a pleasure to see that he had been freed up to become a man.

William said he would come to see me if he got bad again and I said I would be available if he did, but we both knew it wasn't going to happen. Partly because I thought he would be able to manage any minor and temporary re-occurrence, but more because I was a part of a previous life which he had already left behind.

2

George's Bad Back and Accepting the Patient

NOT ALL PATIENTS GET BETTER. NO SYSTEM OF medicine always works. Sometimes the reasons are obvious but more often it is a mystery. What seemed to be a convincing diagnosis didn't produce effective treatments; or the patient appeared to respond well at first but then didn't improve anymore; or some symptoms cleared up but others remained stubbornly resistant to change. I find it immensely frustrating, especially when I have run out of ideas. What then? Do I keep on treating, hoping that all the sessions will have a cumulative effect and that one day they will add up and there will be a sudden breakthrough? Or do I simply say that I have done my best and admit that I cannot help?

George and Rachel spring to mind as soon as I start to think about my failures. With most of the others, and there are quite a few, I feel comfortable simply saying that there was nothing more I could have done and that no system of medicine can guarantee success. But with these two I can't help wondering if I could have done better.

George is retired now. He was a very good violinist who played professionally in a top orchestra and well-known chamber ensembles and he goes to concerts, particularly at the Wigmore Hall, every week. These days he is better known as a master craftsman. With painstaking love and care, and using the finest of materials, he restores old instruments which have been damaged, and after they have been through his hands they sing out once again with a tone as clear and fine as when they were first made. I know that I should treat him just like all my other patients but I have enormous admiration for professional musicians, and for skilled craftsmen too, and as George is both I can't help feeling a little humbled in his presence.

The first thing that struck me about him was the enormous contrast between his face and his posture. His face is thin with very delicate features and deep-set eyes, the face of a monk in a renaissance painting. But whereas the monk might look severe, George's expression is gentle, humorous and kindly; the look of a man who has experienced much in his life and has ended up finding it amusing and delightful.

His posture on the other hand is distressing. He is tall with a pronounced stoop, and his body is bent over to one side. His right shoulder is a good four or five inches higher than his left and it is rolled inwards as well, so he walks in a crab-like way, leading with the right hand side of his body and peering over his shoulder to see where he is going. It looked desperately uncomfortable and I thought he must be in constant pain.

But he didn't start by telling me about his back but about a recent diagnosis of Parkinson's disease. 'It is a terrible blow,' he said. I could well imagine it. 'I dread not having control of my hands,' he went on. 'What am I to do if I can't work? Can't play the violin? Can acupuncture help with Parkinson's?'

This is often a key moment in a first session. Of course patients want a prognosis, but until I have given them a few treatments and seen how they respond I really don't like making any predictions, especially as each patient is unique and each condition is complex. On the other hand, patients do need some information before they start to spend time and money on treatment. And it is also important to make sure that they don't have unreasonable expectations, otherwise they will be quickly disappointed with acupuncture and with me.

'If acupuncture could cure Parkinson's,' I started, 'the world would know all about it, so we can rule that out. What it might be able to do – and this depends on a host of things which I'll talk about in a minute – is to slow down the progress of the disease or even, at best, stop it getting any worse than it is now. But I won't know if that is possible until I've found out a lot more about you and examined you carefully. So let's talk more when I've done that.'

There was no tremor in George's hands, so when I started to check his structure I was expecting to find rigidity – which is the other way the disease manifests. And I did, but somehow it didn't feel systemic. That is, there were places where his musculature was extremely stiff and contracted but there were also plenty of places where it was firm but flexible. As I felt along his torso I puzzled over the difference – why had it hit him in some places and not others? Why that pronounced pulling towards the left? And then I suddenly saw him playing the violin and realised how it twists the body in exactly the way George's body was twisted. Could it be that the distortion in him was not the disease at all but simply the long-term effect of the hours each day on his violin? Or perhaps the disease came in on top of the distortion, so to speak, and had frozen him in the position he had adopted for so long?

I stopped and asked him about his back pain. Indeed it had been creeping up on him for years and indeed it was mainly on the right and in the middle and upper back. I asked if it was common among violinists. 'These days,' he replied, 'all the music colleges teach students to look after their bodies. They have Alexander lessons and all that. But there was nothing of the sort when I was a student, or even a professional musician. And yes, everyone's back hurts. We just thought we had to put up with it.'

I bent down to take his pulses and I went first to the Liver pulse. One function of the Liver, in the words of the ancient texts, is to smooth energy in the body, so any disease that makes a person shake or seize up could well be a Liver issue. The pulse was both floating and wiry, to use traditional descriptions, but in the language with which I tried to express what I was feeling under my fingertips, it was anxious, distressed and tense. All the other pulses had something of the same quality but to a much lesser extent, and the Fire pulses were noticeably weaker than the rest.

I didn't know if this was a common pulse picture in patients with Parkinson's – or indeed if there is such a thing as a common picture with Parkinson's – but I couldn't help wondering what would happen if the obvious stress in the Liver (and to some extent its paired organ, the Gall Bladder) was eased. Might his body let go of some of that distressing tension? Might his spasticity relax? And might that allow in more warmth which, again, might have a softening effect?

So I asked about his life. He lived in a four-storey terraced house in London which he had bought in the 1970s.

'Jolly lucky,' he commented. 'Couldn't possibly afford it now.'

He told me his wife had died twenty years before and he had been on his own ever since; no children. So I asked if he looked after himself properly.

'Oh, yes, I cook a decent meal every evening.'

'And do you sleep well?'

'Well, I do, but it's in two parts, in a sort of a way. I am so tired once I have eaten and it's such a long way upstairs to my bedroom that I often fall asleep at the kitchen table. I wake up in the middle of the night and crawl upstairs, and then I'm usually awake for a bit until I fall asleep again.'

He noticed the expression on my face.

'Bad for my back, do you think?'

'I do.'

He smiled. 'And that's on a good night.' He was teasing me.

'Go on then. Shock me.'

'On a bad night I fall asleep in the bath and when I wake up the water's freezing.'

'I am shocked.'

'You're going to tell me off?' George raised his eyebrows.

'Would it make any difference if I did?'

He nodded. 'No. Quite right. None at all.'

He was enjoying this and so was I, but underneath I was worried. If he carried on abusing his body like this, what chance would I have of making any difference with an hour a week of treatment, at best?

'Any other bad habits I should know about?' I asked.

'Well, it doesn't happen every day, but when I get going with an instrument I get completely engrossed. It's like following a thread through a maze and I can't stop for fear that when I start again I'll have lost the thread. So then I work long hours, can be very long.'

'Where do you do this?'

'I have a workshop. It's about a fifteen-minute walk from home.'

'And do you carry that with you?' I asked, pointing at a large leather bag he had put down on the floor beside him, the kind of bag you imagine Victorian doctors carried about with them.

'Ah. You're going to get disapproving again, I can tell.'

I was about to reply in the same sort of bantering tone but I stopped myself. It was fun batting it back and forth as if we were playing banter tennis, but maybe it wasn't serving him. What attitude should I adopt? What stance should I take? I couldn't tell him off as if he were a little boy. On the other hand I wasn't going to collude in behaviour which could only undermine any treatment.

'It's complicated,' I said. 'I don't know how much is the Parkinson's and how much is the effects of years of violin playing, carrying a heavy bag and falling asleep in the bath; nor do I know how your body will respond to treatment. So I think you should have a few sessions and give me really detailed feedback on the effects of each; then we can decide whether or not it is worth continuing.'

I was pleased to see that he took this seriously. 'Thank you,' he said. 'I thought you were going to throw me out.'

He came weekly after that. The relief he got from the first treatment only lasted a few hours, but by the fourth it held for two or three days. There had been a marked improvement in his posture too and his musculature was much more flexible. So much so that I started to doubt the diagnosis of Parkinson's. Of course I wasn't competent to disagree with his doctors, and I would not do so directly, but I did wonder how he would respond if he were to think that he might not have the disease after all. Some patients go to great lengths to obtain a diagnosis and when they get it they hold on to it as a cherished passport to the realm of the sick. But I didn't think George was like that. I waited to see the results of a couple more sessions, which had the same general effect, and then approached the topic cautiously.

'It's been a pretty good response, don't you think?'

He agreed.

'It may be that treatment is just unravelling the worst of the effects of all those years of distortion – but it may be having a deeper effect too.'

George was as sharp as ever. 'Are you saying you think it has slowed the Parkinson's?'

'It's only guesswork, but yes, I am beginning to think that. But in a way, it'll never be clear because...'

'Because you won't know the difference between a really slow Parkinson's and no Parkinson's at all.'

'Exactly.'

'Not that the distinction makes any difference to me.'

'I suppose that's right.'

'So it's not worth bothering about.'

I wasn't sure that was true but, as so often with George, I couldn't think of a good reply on the spur of the moment.

I carried on treating him weekly for some months but then it became clear that the improvement had stopped. I had to broach the topic which he always managed to avoid.

'I'm not sure treatment is really helping,' I started.

George smiled at me to soften his words. 'Are you threatening to throw me out again?'

'No, of course not.'

'In that case you're going to tell me off, aren't you?'

'I am.' We knew each other well enough by now. 'You've got to start helping yourself. I know it would be a big job moving your bedroom downstairs, but surely you can get someone to help you do it? And it's ridiculous carrying that heavy bag to and fro all the time. It really doesn't help. Can't you leave your stuff in the workshop at the end of the day?'

'No. It's too precious. And the place isn't secure. I wouldn't be able to sleep for worrying about it.'

'Well, get a rucksack. A proper, modern, well-designed one. Then at least the weight would be properly distributed onto your hips. Then it would help your back to straighten up rather than being pulled down by that bag.'

George looked shocked. 'One of those ones ramblers use?'

'That's right.'

'I'd look ridiculous.'

I hadn't thought of that. George always looked like a well-dressed man of the 1950s: polished shoes, trousers with a knife-edged crease, sports jacket, tie, trilby, and in winter a practically full-length belted woollen coat.

'It won't quite go with your outfit, I grant you that, but who cares?'

'I care.'

'Wouldn't you rather get better?'

'Are you guaranteeing that if I wear a rucksack' – he drawled out the word 'rucksack' as if it were some foul, evil-smelling blockage in a drain – 'I'll get better?'

'Of course I can't guarantee it. You know I can't.'

I suddenly realised what I was up against. I'd always known that George was clever and that if he chose to argue with me he would find ways of slipping away from what I was trying to say. But for the first time I saw an implacable stubbornness. He was not going to stop carrying that bag, nor was he going to stop working very long hours hunched over a workbench, nor would he stop falling asleep at the kitchen table and nor would he move his bedroom down from the top floor. Of course, in the end, he was entitled to live the way he wanted – but where did that leave me? And where did it leave his treatment?

I had become very fond of George. What's more, I cared that he could go on playing his violin and mending instruments for people to play and enjoy, but could I honestly carry on if I thought there was no realistic prospect of the treatments doing any good? On the other hand, could I really throw him out – to use his phrase – if he wanted to keep coming?

As I worried about what to do I remembered that I had come across something similar once before, so I went and looked back at my notes to see if I had come up with a solution then.

Rachel was a remarkable mathematician. She had won every possible prize at school and at university and then went to work for one of the biggest of the merchant banks at an eye-watering salary. By the time she was thirty-two, when she came to see me, she had developed a particular expertise which was so uncommon and so vital to the bank that she could practically name her price.

She had found a method of assessing and evaluating risk and with it had steered the bank into investments which no one else would take on but which turned out to be hugely profitable, and away from others which looked good but weren't.

However, her employer had its own risk to assess. Rachel had fallen out with the first bank that had taken her on straight from university, and was now causing trouble in her second. She was so used to being right in her mathematical work, it seemed, that she thought she was right about everything else as well. So when the bank made big decisions which she thought were wrong she had no hesitation in telling colleagues, directors, even clients, how stupid they were. What's more, she seemed to insist on arguing with everyone, even with those who actually agreed with her. The head of human resources kept telling her to calm down and toe the line but it made no difference at all. Finally the bank decided that she was more trouble than she was worth and gave her a large sum of money to go away.

She took the news calmly, assuming she would immediately walk into another job. But her work was very specialised and only relevant to a small number of organisations and by now she had a reputation for being extremely difficult, so although she had applied for a number of jobs she hadn't had a single interview.

She came to me complaining of a bad back but that didn't seem to bother her as much as the long list of small symptoms she told me about each time, hardly any of which were the same each time and hardly any of which could possibly be amenable to acupuncture – or indeed any form of medicine. Throughout each session she hardly stopped talking, asking me question after question about acupuncture and bodywork, intelligent penetrating questions, but ones which I had only just started to answer before she would start to ask the next one. I found it exhausting trying to keep up with her. Then, just as she was leaving and just as I had stopped thinking about her and had started to put away my notes, she would pause with her hand on the doorknob and tell me of some symptom which was far more important than any of the ones she had mentioned in the treatment – and then ask if there was anything I could do to help with it.

It was frustrating; and it was also frustrating that I couldn't work out what was causing her back pain. Usually, by palpation, I can find where energy is blocked and usually, then, I can work out how best to relieve the blockage so that relief and healing can follow. But with Rachel I couldn't feel blocked energy under my hands, nor any distortion in the structure of the spine, nor indeed unusual tension in a particular muscle group. So I tried different things in each treatment hoping that, sooner or later and more by luck than judgement, I would find something that worked. Meanwhile, Rachel continued to come almost weekly.

I thought a good deal about whether or not I should continue to treat her. Normally, I do not continue if I see no signs of change. But with Rachel it occurred to me that after such a glittering start to her career she must find it unbearable that it had all crashed so badly and that perhaps the only way this distress could manifest was by physical pain and niggles, cramps and stiffnesses.

I remembered a passage from a book by an eminent neurologist:

> I have met many people whose sadness is so overwhelming that they cannot bear to feel it. In its place they develop physical disabilities. Against all logic, people's subconscious selves choose to be crippled by convulsions or wheelchair-bound rather than experience the anguish that exists inside them... I have found myself astounded by the degree of disability that can arise as a result of psychosomatic illness. (O'Sullivan 2015, p.15)

Rachel's ailments weren't as serious as these but I thought that might be what was happening, and that treatment might allow her to feel her distress rather than develop symptoms in its place.

We carried on with treatment for almost a year but nothing happened and nothing changed. Each time she came she would report much the same pain in her back and would read out her list of minor symptoms. I started to feel uncomfortable. Perhaps I was colluding in some fantasy of hers? Perhaps I was playing a part in keeping her stuck? For I could imagine her thinking that as she came for treatment almost every week she was doing all she could to be well, whereas the treatment might actually be a substitute for what she really needed to do. I could imagine myself in three or four years' time greeting Rachel as she turned up at my treatment room as if I were the waiter in her favourite café, part of a routine, even a ritual, which occupied her time but made absolutely no difference to her health.

And then I came across the following sentence: 'We are on a perilous margin when we begin to look passively at our future selves, and see our own figures led with dull consent into insipid misdoing and shabby achievement' (Eliot 1994[1871–2], p.783). It seemed to fit me exactly, so at her next appointment I told Rachel that I didn't think I was helping as her symptoms had not improved for quite some time, and suggested she go instead to a cranial osteopath for whom I have great respect.

'But you're the only person I can talk to.' There was hostility in her eyes, not pleading.

'If it's talking you want then you should go to a psychotherapist – I'm not trained.' As the words came out of my mouth I could hardly believe I hadn't said it long before. It seemed so obvious, now, that it was what she really needed.

'But there's nothing wrong with me.'

'There's something wrong with all of us,' I replied. 'That's not the point. The point is that it is terribly frustrating for you not to have work that uses that enormous brain of yours. And it's a waste too. Talking it all through with someone properly trained might help you to see things differently and find ways of changing the situation you are in.'

'You don't understand. I don't have to "change the situation I'm in"' – she said these words with heavy sarcasm. 'The people in the banks've got it in for me and they've all agreed to blacklist me.'

'That might be true. If so, that is precisely the situation you are in, and you won't change it by changing them.'

'You don't understand.'

'Maybe not. In that case I'm no use to you.'

'Damn right you're not.' And she slammed out of the room.

That was more than five years before, but as I read my notes I remembered the regret I felt at the time about the way this had ended. Could I do better with George?

I tried framing the problem in a number of ways, but I ended up thinking that any treatment I could devise would be defeated by George's determination not to change the way he lived. I was sympathetic – none of us finds it easy to admit that we can no longer go on doing what we want to do in the way we want to do it. So possibly the way to reach George was to point out that it was a matter of choice. He could continue as he was but the damage it was doing would mean that before long he wouldn't be able to go to his beloved concerts, and before long he would be unable to look after himself; and I couldn't imagine George taking kindly to being in a home of some sort. Didn't he want to postpone these things for as long as possible?

He didn't. When I put it to him he smiled and said, 'Good of you to give me the option but I choose to stay as I am.'

After he left I sat there for a while wondering if I could go on treating him when I could see no prospect of success. Was I wasting his time and money? Was it the same as with Rachel, who wasn't going to get better either? Somehow I felt it was different but I couldn't see why. That evening, mulling it all over, I became clear that I was willing to carry on with George even though I knew he wasn't going to get better, but I hadn't been willing with Rachel – what was the difference between them?

The question made me think of another patient, one who had also turned up every few weeks with small but apparently annoying symptoms: a big toe that hurt occasionally, a twitch in his left eye one day, a cramp he got at night in his calf muscles and so on. At some point, and I don't really know why, I found myself asking him if he was interested in all these symptoms.

'Not particularly,' he replied. 'Why do you ask?'

'Well, it seems as if you are. Quite a lot of them are very temporary and yet you describe them in as much detail as if they were long-standing problems. So I thought perhaps you took an interest, maybe even enjoyed talking about them to someone.' Behind this, although I did not mean it unkindly, was the clear implication that many of the things he brought for treatment he could really just ignore. To my surprise not only did he pick up the implication of what I was saying, he became animated for the first time. He sat up in his chair, he waved his arms about and he spoke with gusto.

'You're right, you're right! It's true. It's because I've got to have something to talk about with someone intelligent. You have no idea how dull my life is. I didn't realise quite how dull it's been since I retired. Dull, dull.' He seemed to like the sound of the word. 'Dull. Oh God! My wife's friends are so dull, and they are the only ones we see. All mine were from work and they live miles away or I've lost touch. So it's taking the dog for a walk every morning, picking up a grandchild from school on Tuesday, bridge on Wednesday, tennis on Friday, people for dinner on Saturday, all the same people, all of them ghastly. You've no idea. And these symptoms, they're dull too, no wonder you're not interested – how could you possibly be? I can't imagine how you manage to pay attention to me droning on about them every time I see you. Well, I'll stop it. Quite right. Get a grip.'

So I gave him a completely different treatment from before. I ignored all his symptoms and just did points which would stimulate him, get things moving, bring in a breath of fresh air. By agreement we made another appointment in two months' time rather than two weeks, and when we next met he had bought a horse and was riding every day. 'I loved riding when I was younger and I was good at it. So I've taken it up again and I love it.'

'Not dull?' I teased him.

After that he came twice a year, regular as clockwork. 'Like going to the dentist,' he said.

And I saw that, like George but unlike Rachel, he was willing to be truthful about himself and his life. It didn't matter that he had embraced change while George had refused to do so; what mattered is that each of them was willing to own up to what they were like and decide either to change or to take the consequences. But Rachel was not willing to do so and that was why the treatments were never going to work.

So the next time I saw George I told him that I would carry on treating him for as long as he wanted. He looked at me quizzically and said, 'Lucky I am a good bit older than you.' I smiled, and agreed that it might take me well beyond retiring age. But then, when he had disarmed me, he added, 'I wondered if you would ever accept me as I am.'

It landed like a blow. That was why he had often talked about me throwing him out. He had sensed, quite rightly, that I hadn't accepted him as he was. And I saw that I could not help him, nor indeed anyone else, unless I was able to do just that.

3

Stacey's Strange Symptoms and Psychosomatic Illness

LIKE MOST ACUPUNCTURISTS I SEE A LOT OF STRANGE symptoms: a young woman who has had a permanent deep ache in one buttock for the past ten years; a man who keeps falling because, as he told me, 'the right hand side of my body digs its heel in'; a woman who always wakes at two in the morning and can only go back to sleep again if she eats cheese. Many patients come to acupuncturists because their doctors have been unable to help; they don't have any identifiable disease and their blood tests have shown nothing unusual.

Stacey was one of these patients. A physiotherapist in her mid thirties, she was an endurance athlete, super fit, very strong, and a keen rock climber, so it was no surprise when she told me that she specialised in treating sports injuries. She worked as a busy independent practitioner, and a top professional rugby club called her in when one of their players wasn't responding well enough to the care of their in-house practitioner. In other words she was really good at her job.

Because of her training Stacey had a thorough knowledge of anatomy and a deep appreciation of Western medicine, so when she started to get odd bouts of acute pain in the top of her chest on the left, pain which radiated to the throat and shoulder, she was pretty sure she had a heart problem and took herself off for the appropriate tests. They all came back clear. As far as any of her doctors could tell there was absolutely nothing wrong with her heart; on the contrary, all its functions were working exceptionally well. The only two explanations they could offer for the sudden pains were, firstly, that they might be muscular spasms, and she knew enough about her body to be pretty sure that wasn't the cause, or secondly some kind of virus in her system whose activity was normally suppressed but which could affect her when she was tired or run down.

Well, at least it was a theory, but the next few times the pain hit her she found that it happened when she was feeling well, neither tired nor run down. She started to get worried. Should she give up climbing? After all, she couldn't imagine how she would cope if it were to happen on a rock face. And was there some lingering disease process going on in her which, if left untreated, might lead to disability or worse? What's more, after a few months she started to get new symptoms. If she started to feel dizzy she knew that the pain would hit her within the next twenty-four hours. Then, when it did, although it was just as acute as before, now it jumped her heart rate to almost double its normal sixty a minute. Also, when it first started she felt fine again as soon as the pain had stopped, but now it could take as much as two days for her heart rate to return to normal, and until it did so she had to struggle to breathe properly. She couldn't work and had to cancel all her patients for the next couple of days.

Our first session was awkward. She seemed ill at ease, as if going to an acupuncturist was slightly shameful for her, like resorting to the services of a quack. I didn't much care for the role nor for the way she stressed that she had only come because her mother, whom I had treated in the past, insisted that she saw me. I did think of refusing to take her on as a patient. I didn't mind if she didn't believe in acupuncture – that doesn't get in the way of it working; after all, vets use it on their patients, and presumably the cats and dogs, the horses and cows, have no strong opinions about it either way. And in any case one of the most successful courses of treatment I ever gave was to a tall, wild Irishman, who, when he arrived in the clinic waiting room, would announce in a booming voice to all those present, 'I don't believe in any of this malarkey, you know.' No, the problem with Stacey was that I suspected she had turned up simply because she wanted to get her mother off her back – so she could say to her, 'Well, I went and saw him and he stuck pins in me and it didn't work – so stop going on at me about it.' In other words, although I don't mind patients not believing in acupuncture, I do mind them coming in order to prove it doesn't work. That becomes self-fulfilling.

But I was interested in Stacey's strange symptoms, I cared that she could continue do the work and the sport she loved, and I thought there was at least a chance I could help. It isn't easy to say exactly why I thought that, but looking back on it, and on plenty of other similar examples too, I think it's when I sense some strong disturbance in the patient's energy. If that disturbance were to be cleared, I suppose I think to myself, then there is a good chance that the symptoms will resolve too. If, on the other hand, I can't see anything obvious that I could start to change with my needles, then what could I possibly gain by sticking them in?

With Stacey what was noticeable – no, it was more than that – what was striking was the contrast between this tall, fit young woman with a powerful presence and the fact that she didn't seem to inhabit her body. She spoke, she smiled, she nodded, but she was like a rather bad actor playing the part of Stacey. I found that I didn't quite believe what she was saying nor what she was communicating non-verbally; the words were too bland, the smile too superficial, the gestures too robotic. Who is she, I found myself wondering, and what is going on inside?

So I thought I would give her one treatment. If nothing happened then she could go back to her mother with her prepared speech; but if there was enough change to persuade her to have more treatment then perhaps I could really help. I thought it was a chance worth taking. At the time it seemed like a reasonable plan but it ignored two things. One was my initial doubt about treating her – an intuition and perhaps an accurate one; and the other was the question of how far I was willing to go to support her.

With most patients it isn't hard to judge how much they might need. If someone arrives for a first treatment with a serious illness or disability then I know that I might be working with them for years. It is a big commitment and I don't take it on lightly. But usually people turn up with conditions which I expect to get better quite quickly and easily; and if they don't then the two of us usually agree it isn't worth persisting. So I don't have to think all that carefully about accepting them as patients. Looking back on it, I should have realised that Stacey didn't really fit into either of these categories, so I didn't know what I was letting myself in for.

By the time we'd talked about her symptoms and their history and I'd gathered some other basic information about her life and health, there wasn't a great deal of time left for needling, so I did something very simple – three points only and all based on one single idea: that perhaps her lack of presence was a lack of the kind of energy that warms a person. I couldn't help thinking of a central heating boiler that has gone out. It still hangs on the wall but it isn't doing anything, and more specifically it isn't heating anything. So I needled three basic Fire points. Very simple. I usually do something simple at first, partly so I can assess the effect of the needles and partly in case my initial diagnosis is wrong – at least then the patient won't have to live with an energy system which has been badly distorted by my work. I often think of these first points as me saying to the patient's body, and unconscious mind, 'Hello. How do you feel about this? Are you interested in changing?'

Stacey phoned me the next morning. She told me she had had a terrible time since the treatment. She had become jumpy and irritable, had hardly slept that night, and when she did she had appalling nightmares in which everybody got killed. She was feeling too vulnerable to go to work, so could she come and see me, please, and get put back to where she was? I said I was sorry it had been so difficult and booked her in at the end of the day – the first space I had.

I watched her park the car – when she arrived the day before I was with another patient and I had missed it. It was fascinating. She reversed into a space which was about as wide and as deep as two cars, so she had plenty of room. Given her phone call I thought she might make a bit of a mess of it. On the contrary, she did it perfectly, putting her car exactly in the middle, first time. But that clearly wasn't good enough. She sat in the car looking around her, deciding whether or not to try again. Then she got out and had another look, front and back. She must have come to the conclusion that it wasn't quite right as she got back in the car, started the engine, moved back about a foot, maybe two; handbrake on, looked around again, got out and checked again. Finally, this time, she seemed satisfied. She locked the car carefully, checking the handle afterwards, and walked towards me. So she didn't seem like the distraught person she had described on the phone and nor was she quite like the person I met yesterday. It was a bit of a puzzle.

'I didn't know what to expect,' she said as she sat down, 'but it certainly wasn't that.'

'I know.' My tone was conciliatory. 'The first time you never quite know what's going to happen.'

'Can you undo it? I can't function like this.'

'I think if you had no more treatment you'd just go back to where you were, and quite quickly too. Yesterday obviously had a big effect, though I doubt it'll last long. But if I do another treatment it will carry on the change that has just started. So you have to choose, really, whether you want to go back to where you were, in which case I won't treat you again, or whether you want to change.'

She thought for a moment and then said, 'I thought it would be gradual.'

Of course! Because that is the way she gets fit. She builds up carefully, pushing herself a little more each day, each week, each month. And that is how she works with her own patients, giving them exercises to increase their mobility bit by bit. She has no experience or understanding of an energetic change – which can indeed be sudden and chaotic.

'It's sometimes gradual,' I said, 'but it looks as though it might be a bumpy ride for you.'

'Why's that? Why would it be?' she asked.

I didn't know, of course. Why indeed had it been so disturbing for her? When I have no real explanation I reach for an analogy – and ideally one which will speak to the patient's experience. 'Ever been canoeing?' I asked. 'White water?' She nodded. 'Well,' I continued, 'you paddle along for a bit and it's all smooth and straightforward. Then you come to the rapids and it's chaos. You get tossed and turned and hurled about and you might capsize, and then you come out of it and it's all smooth and straightforward again. Well, it's like that. Big changes, like a change in the level of the river, tend to be chaotic.'

She nodded again. The analogy made sense to her and for the first time I felt some connection between us.

'As a matter of fact,' she said somewhat shamefacedly, 'it wasn't so smooth before.'

The atmosphere in the room changed, as it always seems to do when the truth is being told. It goes still, somehow, and charged. I often find myself holding my breath so as not to disturb it, not wanting it to drop back into the normal and the mundane.

'Oh?' I looked enquiringly at her. Here it comes, I thought, the story she hasn't told me. But she didn't rise to the bait. 'Could we do one more then?' she asked. 'See how it goes?' She was like a nervous swimmer, dipping her toe in cold water and wondering whether or not to take the plunge.

Why should I insist that she jumps in? I asked myself. Is she not entitled to take her time? Do I need to know what has been going wrong in her life? Can I not just give her a treatment and hope that it helps?

I think that's when I knew that Stacey was going to be a challenge. But I also recognised that she was making as big a commitment as she could. I decided to acknowledge that by doing the same.

When she lay down on the couch this time I thought I would palpate the areas where she had pain because I get so much diagnostic information through touch. I asked her if it would be alright if I put my hands on her upper chest on the left, above the breast, and she agreed. It was a strange sensation. The strength and solidity of her pectoral muscles was remarkable, but even more remarkable was that they seemed to shrink or wither under my hands. It was almost as if she was trying to escape my attention, to hide away and go somewhere deeper where she could not be found. I took my hands off, went and made a note, and then tried again. Yes, there it was. Not as clear as before but definitely the same movement away from me.

By now I was pretty sure of the diagnosis. It is not one which makes any sense in Western medicine, but then Stacey's symptoms didn't make any sense in Western medicine. It is well known in many pre-modern medical traditions such as herbalism, shamanism and acupuncture, and they all have treatments for it; in fact even the Christian church has a treatment for it. It has many different names and many different causes are attributed to it, but they all amount to the same thing: that something alien was in her and needed to be removed. That was what I was feeling under my hands and that was what I sensed early on, when I found myself wondering who she was and where she was.

I put the needles in and sat back and waited. Sometimes the effect is dramatic; sometimes nothing much seems to happen. But when it is working there is usually a change in the pulses, in the expression in the patient's eyes and most of all in the atmosphere in the room. It feels lighter, and the air seems easier to breathe. Imagine a room in a damp humid place, perhaps in an old house by a river on a rainy summer's evening; now think of being in an upstairs room in a chalet in Switzerland on a clear spring morning – that sort of difference.

It took about ten minutes before I became aware of a change in the room. I got up and checked her pulses and they were better, and so was her skin tone. After another ten minutes I added one more needle, to give the treatment an extra shove. I took the needles out after about half an hour and she got up off the couch looking better, clearer, as if a layer of grime had been wiped off her face.

I said all the usual things about taking care of herself for a little while after the treatment, and I told her she could phone or email if she had any questions or worries. As I said these formal words, words I have said a thousand times or more, a voice inside me said, 'So that'll be tomorrow, then.'

It was tomorrow, and it was the phone, and it was nine o'clock in the morning. Could I see her today? The old symptoms had returned with renewed ferocity – the pain, the breathlessness, the very fast heart rate, the anxiety. And now there was a new symptom – she had spent most of the night vomiting.

For the most part I heard the news with equanimity. I had long since come to the conclusion that the cause of Stacey's problems lay deep, so I wasn't surprised that, once again, she had had a strong reaction to the treatment. But I would be lying if

I said I wasn't a bit worried too. Was I making her worse? Had I started her on a journey she wasn't willing to complete – and if so, what sort of shape would she be in if she stopped before the end? The treatments had clearly woken something which, until then, had only broken into consciousness in the form of the strange symptoms – how would she cope if she really saw and understood it?

It is very rare indeed that I treat someone more than once a week and this was going to be Stacey's third treatment in three days. But I was cheered when I saw her, partly because she looked different again, so something was working, and partly because of what she said as soon as she sat down.

'I feel as if you've stirred up a wasp inside me and it's buzzing and angry.'

'Well, that's a good sign,' I said.

'It is?'

'I think so, yes.'

'Why?'

'Well, instead of being stuck inside you, whatever it was that was causing those strange symptoms of yours is now on the move, so we can help it to leave. Like trapping a wasp in a glass and then letting it fly off outside.'

I didn't add that it was another good sign that she had identified the wasp. It meant that, for the first time, whatever had caused her symptoms was starting to come up to consciousness, where it could be dealt with.

I put the needles in. While there aren't exactly points for trapping wasps and putting them outside, the general idea was clear enough, and there are certainly plenty of points which release pathogens which have become lodged in the body.

After about ten minutes I took her pulses again. She opened her eyes and looked up at me. 'I think it's about Den,' she said.

'Tell me about Den.'

It turned out that Den was a man with whom she had fallen very deeply in love. It was a wildly passionate, sexual relationship and she had never experienced anything like it before. After three weeks, and at her urging, he moved in with her. All went well for a few months but then he started coming home late, and when she asked where he had been, he refused to give any explanation. To cut a long story short it turned out that he was deeply involved in dealing drugs and in organised prostitution. After a day of enormous rows he had walked out, taking with him some of her prize possessions.

'And that's when the chest pain started?'

'Yes.' She was crying now.

'Well, no wonder.'

I kept thinking of a couple of lines of a poem:

In the deserts of the heart
Let the healing fountain start.
(Auden 1976[1947], p.249)

After a while she said, 'Underneath, I'm quite well.'

'I'm sure you are,' I replied.

I treated Stacey five times in seven days – a record which I hope will never be beaten – and then twice more in the following month. She was wobbly and had bad days, but it was clear to us both that, in effect, she was recuperating from a long illness. We used to joke that she ought to be in a convalescent home, sitting in the grounds in a bath chair and having blankets tucked in around her knees.

Stacey had always made appointments on the phone and one day I realised that she hadn't called for a few weeks – and she never did again. I don't know what happened to her, but I suspect she simply went back to being who she was before Den.

Stacey had been deeply affected by an intimate connection to someone who was content to take advantage of human vulnerability and frailty and prosper from it. While Western medicine has deep knowledge of contagion by germs and viruses, it overlooks this kind of contagion.

Stacey's experience and her symptoms were unusual, and unusually severe, but I see the same thing in a much milder form over and over again. So often the root cause of a patient's illness only becomes clear weeks or months after he or she first comes for treatment, and the two of us realise that it started with some emotional shock, some deep disappointment, some injury to the self. When I was a child this kind of idea would have been dismissed as 'psychosomatic illness' – a label which essentially meant that the patient was making it up. We know better now. We live at a time when a famous cancer surgeon can write:

> Years of experience have taught me that cancer and indeed nearly all diseases are psychosomatic. This may sound strange to people accustomed to thinking that psychosomatic ailments are not truly 'real', but believe me they are...the first step is understanding – without guilt or self pity – how the mind has contributed to the body's ills. (Siegel 1990, pp.111–112)

Although there are plenty of doctors who accept these ideas, they lack the kinds of treatments which acupuncturists use all the time. I think of them as catching Stacey's inner wasp and letting it fly away.

Reflections on William, George and Stacey

In spite of the differences between these patients, the basic approach to their treatment was the same for all three of them. There were blockages in the normal flows and circulation of energy in their bodies which were stopping them from re-gaining their health – so the goal of treatment was simply to remove the blockages. With William and Stacey the job was straightforward, at least in principle, because they both turned out to be good examples of well-known diagnoses and well-understood treatments. Most work of most practitioners is like this, and it is good medicine.

But George showed up one of its limitations. Certainly the distortions in his back were severe, but there are plenty of classic diagnoses and treatments for back pain and they have worked for countless patients. So why not for George? Why was he different from the others?

According to Western medicine, the structural distortions in George's back would inevitably cause pain. But a doctor came to understand that this is not necessarily true:

> The speaker after me gave a fascinating lecture on the lack of correlation between the subjective experience of back pain and

the objective measures of musculoskeletal dysfunction, such as X rays and MRI scans. He showed X rays and scans of patients that looked so awful that you could not believe these people could stand or walk, yet they were free of pain and had normal mobility. In other cases, people were immobilised by pain yet their spines looked normal. (Weil 2008[1995], p.120)

The explanation is that we feel pain when energy is not flowing properly through bones and joints. So if energy is going nicely along the curves of a distorted spine then the chances are it won't hurt; and similarly, if energy is not flowing straight down a straight spine, that will probably cause pain or dysfunction. Acupuncture can change the flows of energy so they match the structure properly, and that is how it works to relieve back pain.

For both William and Stacey the blockage in their normal energy flow was caused by a specific trauma and persisted simply because nothing had happened to remove it. But that was not true of George. The existing flows in his back were held in place by his implacable will not to change, and so no change was possible. My time with him helped me to recognise one of the limits of acupuncture. Some blocks are so strong or so ingrained that it would take a miracle to shift them. And similarly, if the patient is committed to staying the same and resisting change, then there is nothing I can do either. It is not my job to force a person to be well if he or she doesn't want to be, and in any case no acupuncture treatment can over-ride a patient's will.

I also learned from these three patients that I cannot dictate or predict what will happen in treatment. William's response was immediately and obviously benign, and with regular acupuncture over a few months he made steady progress to health. Stacey, by contrast, needed five treatments in a week and her journey through them was chaotic. I have no idea why there was that difference between them. And long after it had become clear that I was wrong, I continued to think that George would relent one day and start to take my advice.

All this changed my perception of my work as an acupuncturist. If, as I was taught, I was trying to bring about a particular outcome – a normal bowel for William or the end of Stacey's strange symptoms – then I might easily take the credit if treatment was a success and take the blame if it wasn't. But if, on the other hand, I was simply removing a block then I wouldn't know what might happen afterwards, and the only criterion of success or failure was simply whether or not I had removed the block. Of course I would hope that the patient got better as a result, but that wasn't up to me. Indeed, there was a kind of arrogance in thinking that it might be; there were a thousand other factors and influences on their lives, none of which I could control. So, thanks to my experience with William, I gave up taking both the credit for successes and the blame for failures.

This made such an enormous difference. Instead of trying to force something to happen with stress and effort, I was working instead with a sense of curiosity, fascinated to see what, previously prevented, might now become possible. I had an expertise, it was true, but it was a quite limited one, so I didn't feel removed from my patient by knowing all about how treatment would affect them while they didn't. I began to find the work much easier and my relationships with my patients became more equal. And I am certain that it made me a better practitioner.

And then there was George, who wasn't going to benefit from acupuncture or anything else, as far as I could tell. What did I learn from him? It seems ironic, but I learnt about commitment. Ironic because I suppose I assumed I would feel the most commitment to a patient who was struggling with severe symptoms and a difficult life and for whom I managed to find unlikely but brilliant treatments: but no, I felt it for a patient who had decided not to do what was needed in order to get better and for whom my work made precious little difference. But that was the point. It is the patient who is entitled to decide whether or not treatment is helpful. So once I was committed then I couldn't, in George's phrase, throw him out, as long as he wanted to come. And for all I knew, I realised one day, there might be healing of some sort happening in our sessions even though his back continued to deteriorate.

This thought led me to one last reflection on my work with these patients. The moment William started to laugh my instinct told me that he would get well; with Stacey I found, without actually deciding to do so, that I was willing to treat her more intensively than anyone before or since; and with George I suddenly thought one day that his back might not be the real issue and that treatment might have some other purpose for him. In all three instances, then, I was a bit surprised by my actions and decisions, for they seemed to be more instinctive and intuitive than I was used to. And it occurred to me that it might be precisely through such insights and intuitions that I could do my best work.

4

Sean's Hypochondria and Changing Old Habits

I WAS IMMEDIATELY ATTRACTED TO SEAN. I SUPPOSE you could say it was because he was good-looking and had an instant charm, but neither of these things usually appeal to me particularly, so I thought I must be picking up on something else. It nagged away at the back of my mind for the whole of our first session together and it was only long after he had gone that I managed to put my finger on it. I realised that he was a seeker. He wanted to discover and to understand – and that interested me. So as he greeted me that first time I realised, unconsciously, that he had come to learn. He was forty-two and I was plenty old enough to be a father figure of some sort.

As he walked to my treatment room I noticed he was holding his tall thin body awkwardly, a bit like a stick insect with arthritis. And although he was a good six inches taller than me, when he sat down in his chair – perhaps slumped down would be more accurate – his head was distinctly lower than mine. This was not a man who was comfortable in his body.

An impression that was confirmed when he started to tell me what had brought him for treatment, for there was a long list of symptoms which appeared to be completely unrelated. He had a very itchy scalp and the skin flaked badly; he had recurrent back pain which was sometimes low down and sometimes between the shoulder blades; he had discomfort and restricted movement in his left hip, which had never been quite right since he had keyhole surgery there; he had panic attacks which, though infrequent, were alarming; he sometimes felt dizzy for no reason; he had tremendous problems with his diet and had cut out yeast, sugar, mushrooms and most dairy products but he still got allergic-type reactions to food.

'That's quite a lot of symptoms,' I said. 'Must make life quite difficult.'

'Well, it used to be tricky, but not now, not really.' And he went into a long explanation of how he had been wild when he was young, had partied too hard, had taken too many drugs, but then, just before his fortieth birthday, had gone on a two-week course in America. 'It taught a method of self-discovery. It was wonderful. That's when I found my true self. So, since I've known why I am here on this planet, the physical stuff hasn't bothered me the way it used to. I've got a purpose in life.'

'Oh. And what's that?'

'To tell people about self-discovery.'

Sincerity shone out of him as he said this, but there was something about it all which didn't quite add up. For one thing, he looked a good deal younger than forty-two, and after all that hard living I would have expected him to look older. And then I couldn't quite understand why, if he really wasn't troubled by his symptoms, he had driven more than forty minutes to see me; nor why, if he had found such mental and spiritual contentment, his body was still displaying so many signs of distress. And finally, I usually find that apparently disparate symptoms are at least related, and most often that they all come from one source, but I couldn't see a common theme in Sean's symptoms.

I decided to ask questions about his childhood. In the moment it was an instinctive choice, but looking back on it I suppose I was drawn to the idea because of something boyish about him. And indeed his childhood had been more than difficult: an alcoholic father who left his mother in the lurch; two years in care, along with his two younger siblings; a period of being bullied at school; getting in with what he called the wrong crowd when he was a teenager; and then his first love, a woman he adored, went off with his best friend, so he lost the two most important people in his life at the same time.

'How did you cope between then and now?' I asked.

'Mainly partying, and drugs. I went to Hawaii and got casual work there on building sites. I only came back home two years ago.'

'Did you have all these symptoms when you were there?'

'Not really. A bit. But I didn't pay much attention.'

'So it's since you found your true self that you've been unwell.'

'I suppose it is.' A long pause. 'I hadn't thought of it like that.'

I could see Sean pondering the notion. He didn't speak, and I didn't interrupt the process. Finally he looked up at me and said, 'Do you think my true self is unwell? Is that what you're saying?'

There was nothing combative about his question; he really wanted to know what I thought. Mentally, I took my hat off to him, for he was willing to be challenged – and that is rare in my experience.

'Not at all,' I said. 'I am sure your true self is entirely well. But perhaps the partying and the drugs suppressed your true illnesses as well as your true self – and once you stopped doing all that then both of them came to the surface together.'

Again he thought for a while. And as I waited I found myself looking forward to working with him. I was almost certain that these pauses for thought were windows of opportunity. It had not occurred to him before that his symptoms might have had their origin in the experiences of his early life and that they were now ripe for healing, but there was no resistance, no denial. On the contrary, he was listening; and not just to me, I thought, but to the promptings of some inner voice.

Suddenly, and for the first time, Sean looked at me directly. 'I want to get well. Are you saying these things I've told you about aren't really physical problems? Do you think I have to go to a therapist and talk through it all? Are you telling me you can't help?'

Good questions. If his symptoms were psychosomatic, at least to some extent, then it was reasonable to wonder whether or not acupuncture was appropriate. In my opinion, and as the word 'psychosomatic' suggests, symptoms like his can be relieved through work on the psyche or work on the body – he could choose either approach. I told him that, and added a bit more: 'It's also the fact that acupuncture, like all forms of energy medicine, doesn't draw a hard and fast line between what is mental and what is physical – as Western medicine does. A good acupuncture treatment should make a difference to all of you; you should have fewer symptoms, they should be less severe, and you may view your illnesses and your life rather differently. As to which comes first, or which has the greater effect – who knows? But they do go together.'

He grinned at me, eyebrows raised. 'I like the sound of that.'

I had to make a decision about the first treatment. I could try to do something which I thought would help his main symptom – but which was it? – or try to mobilise his own natural capacity for healing. The latter seemed to me a clearer idea, so I went about it in the usual way. That is, I took his pulses and looked at his tongue in order to get an overall picture of what was happening; both of them showed plenty of signs of distress. I then asked myself – What would really help Sean? What does he need? I sat and waited for some kind of answer, and what came to me was that he had not had much comfort in his life. Perhaps a very comforting treatment would support him, might suggest that he didn't have to worry so much about his symptoms and give him a bit of breathing space – I had no idea why these words came to me, but as soon as they did I felt that sense of relief which I get when something inside me says I am on the right track.

So I needled what I think of as the most comforting points on the body. He looked better for it, but I knew that I would only find out next time if it was what he really needed.

It was a disappointment. As he stalked down the corridor again and slumped in the chair again, nothing about him seemed to have changed. And when I asked him how he had been since the last treatment and whether he had noticed any difference, he went into a long and detailed account of what seemed to me very minor physical responses. His right shoulder had been not exactly painful, not exactly sore, but he had noticed it didn't feel the same for a few days; there was a new ache in his right calf; his left foot felt odd, as if it was widening; and so on and so on. There was no mention of all the other symptoms, so I went through them one by one and they were all just as before. There was only one thing that gave me any encouragement and that was that he had stopped the car on the way home, slept for an hour and woken up feeling good – and he had never done that in the past after any kind of therapy.

I was faced with a very common dilemma. The first treatment hadn't done much; did that mean I hadn't done enough to make a difference, in which case I needed to do more of the same; or did it mean that my basic approach was wrong? In general I tend to change my approach, but with Sean I felt that he was so starved that it might take a while before he was sufficiently nourished by treatment that he could start to recover. So I did different points but all with the same idea in mind.

And the third time I saw him there was definitely a change. There was more flexibility and fluidity in his body; previously he had either been held tight or collapsed, now he walked more smoothly and sat more upright. And I was heartened too when he told me he had felt 'quite emotional all week' – it seemed like progress compared to the endless detail of the previous time.

'What is the feeling?' I asked, expecting an emotion like grief or sadness. What I got was quite different.

'It's a knot. Here.' He made his hand into a fist and put it on his solar plexus, on the mid line just below the rib cage, a place where there is an acupuncture point which has a deep connection to the heart.

'Anything else about it?'

'It feels like a fire in there.'

I was moved. Of the five phases or elements in Chinese medicine the heart is associated with fire. I took it as a clear message that what was needed was treatment for his heart.

Did that mean my first approach was wrong and I should have been treating his heart all along; or had we got to this point only because of what I did first? I didn't know, and I'll never know. It's terribly frustrating, but it is true of any kind of medicine – you can't go back and see what would have happened if you had made different choices; nor can you start again because the previous treatment will have changed the patient, at least to some extent.

Although I knew I was going to treat the heart, I went through the list of symptoms once again. All more or less the same, except for one thing. He told me that he had relaxed his very rigid diet, and had even had some alcohol for the first time in months.

'How was it?'

'Fine. I thought I might have to pay for it but it was fine.'

'Why did you decide to do it?'

'I don't know. And I don't want to wonder why.'

Well, that was interesting. On the one hand I thought it must be a good thing that he could tolerate more foods, taking it as a sign that treatment was making him more resilient and robust. On the other hand, this was the first time he had turned away from me and my questions. I made no comment, and I certainly wasn't going to push him to talk about it if he didn't want to.

But I thought about it a lot that evening. It could have been good; it could have been that he was feeling better and wanted to stop obsessing, as he surely had done, about his diet and his intolerances, and simply wanted to forget about it all. But it could have been that he had felt pressured into exposing himself, perhaps he felt that he had gone too far in revealing the fire in him and wanted to draw a line, call a halt to the process before it became more intrusive. Again, there was no way of knowing for sure, and again I reflected on how often in the course of treating a patient I have to rely on my instinct, my hunches, my best guesses.

The next time he came there was an enormous change in him. He had lost some of that boyish charm but looked the better for it, I thought – more real. Nor did he have a lot to say. Instead of the endless detail he simply reported that most of his symptoms had improved, and left it at that. But half way through the treatment he opened his eyes, looked up at me and said, 'When I was bullied at school, at break time, I used to go into a hiding place where they couldn't get me. It was on a narrow ledge between two buildings, too narrow for the whole of my feet, so I had to hang on with my arms.' He paused. 'I've been hanging on ever since.'

It was one of those moments when it is a privilege to be with a patient, to be a witness to the truth being told. Then he said, 'I don't have to hang on anymore.'

I thought I might not see him again after that, and indeed it was almost a year before he made another appointment. In the meantime he had been back to Hawaii where he had worked as a life coach, teaching people the method of self-discovery which, in his view, had made such a difference to his life.

And then we were right back to where we had been in his first session almost eighteen months before. There was a long list of apparently unrelated symptoms, some new – 'when I get cold I get a terrible earache' – and some of them old – he was on a very restricted diet again and was losing weight too. He had been to various therapists, some of whom sounded a bit dubious, such as the person who told him, without doing any tests, that he had candida and then sold him two hundred pounds' worth of supplements to cure it. 'Did they work?' I asked. 'Can't say they made any difference,' he replied.

That was also true of the treatments I had given him a year before, I reflected. They might have helped a bit in the short term but the truth was they hadn't shifted him from where he was and they hadn't enabled him to walk the path back to health. As he talked I noticed my attention wandering. I couldn't summon up much interest in the detail of his cold hands and feet or the sour taste in his mouth, so I was wondering whether or not to treat him again. Was I willing to be one of a long line of therapists who had tried and failed? And even if I was willing to persist for as long as it took, was he willing to stick with it? I doubted it. Of course I could feel compassion for a kind and caring man who had had a very hard childhood and who seemed to be stuck with the patterns laid down all that time ago, but as he talked on and on I found myself getting restless, at first, then angry.

Was it because he had effectively rejected the work we had done together, and turned down the opportunity it had opened up? Was I simply offended? Was I feeling that he hadn't appreciated my treatments? They were possibilities alright, for I have felt all these things in the past. But when I asked myself as honestly as I could I didn't get that 'oh yes' inside, which I take as a truthful answer. There was some other explanation.

And as so often, it was obvious once I saw it. I was picking up on his anger. It was he who was angry, not me. And then, just as I saw the anger in him, I heard him say, 'I should be rewarded.' A remarkable phrase, and one which pointed to why he was angry. After all, given such a difficult start in life he had done remarkably well. He had kicked a drug habit, supported himself, found out who he was, at least to his own satisfaction, and helped others do the same; and yet he still couldn't eat what he wanted, still couldn't live without pain and discomfort, still had to drag around to therapist after therapist looking for a cure. And he was furious about it.

I looked at him afresh and I couldn't imagine how I had missed it before. Now I knew, it was unmistakable. He hid it pretty well but still, I thought, that is the difference between me and the great practitioners who had been my teachers; they would have seen it straight away.

And it was that anger, I suspected, which was keeping him stuck. It must have taken enormous amounts of energy to keep it in – I had the image of a large concrete block in his solar plexus, the place where he had put his fist. Of course! A fist. That's for hitting people with. And if so much energy was being used to repress that anger then there would hardly be enough for normal life, let alone for any healing to happen.

So I told him. I started to say that I thought he had to deal with his anger. I had quite a lot more to say about it but he interrupted me immediately.

'I'm not angry.'

'I absolutely understand that you aren't aware of your anger,' I replied, 'but I think it is there all the same, and I think it is at the root of your symptoms.'

He gave me a very sweet smile as he shook his head. He did indeed have a lot of charm. No doubt it had been a great help in his life, but it had also been a great hindrance, for he had come to believe that its warm, friendly and engaging ease was who he was and how he was. His anger had been hidden from him just as it had been hidden from everyone else.

I didn't give him a treatment. For one thing I didn't believe it would do any good, and for another I wanted him to get the message that it was time he started to do some work himself, rather than expecting others to fix all his symptoms. I told him that in my opinion the best thing he could do was to become aware of his anger and to look at it absolutely dispassionately without evaluating or judging it, simply asking questions such as What does it feel like? Where is it in the body? Does it move, and if so, in what direction? What ignites it or calms it? – and so on. I went on to say that I thought that if he were to do that he would learn a lot and, what's more, the symptoms would then reduce, at least.

It was interesting. What had first attracted me to Sean was that he was a seeker, someone committed to finding out about himself and about life, and here he was refusing to look at one of the most basic of emotions, one which we all have even though we may express or repress it in different ways. But then, I reflected, each of us has our blind spots, things we cannot see though they are obvious to others; and opening our eyes to them can be hard and sometimes painful. Instinctively, we have kept these things well out of sight because we sense that we might not be able to cope with what would be revealed if we were to acknowledge them. And so it was with Sean's anger. He had probably assumed, completely unconsciously, that it was so huge and so violent that if he were to allow it out he wouldn't be able to cope.

When I explained what I was thinking he listened politely but showed no interest in what I was saying. Well, I thought, I have to say what I believe, right or wrong; it's all I can do. Then it is up to him. But as we parted I didn't think he would ever come back.

I under-estimated him. It was about four months later that he turned up again. Ostensibly he had come because he had been in a road accident which had shaken him and he wanted me to treat him for shock. But it only took a minute or two before he told me that he had been looking at his anger and it had worked.

'Tell me what "working" means.'

'I enjoyed it.'

'Really?'

'Not at first. It was huge at first, but as I kept on it shrank.'

'Are you still doing it?'

'Not so much, but every now and then. It's still there, but it doesn't have a hold on me.'

It was music to my ears. And I waited with as much patience as I could muster to see if he was going to mention all his symptoms and tell me whether or not they had improved. Then he said, 'By the way, I'm much more relaxed about what I eat and I've put on a fair bit of weight. I used to be so fearful of food and I'm not anymore.'

'That's great,' I said, wondering if he was going to connect it to the awareness of his anger.

'Oh, and the itchy scalp is better too.'

'Good.'

'And being cold all the time.'

'Good.'

It went on like this for some time. Is he teasing me, I wondered? Is he deliberately holding back the punchline? No, he wasn't. He finished the list and all his symptoms had improved, but he still said nothing about the attention he had paid to his anger and the role it might have played in all this. Was I waiting because I needed him to acknowledge what I had done, and to say how brilliant I had been to suggest it? Probably. So I just gave it up and said, 'I'd keep on looking at your anger, if I were you. I think you can get more out of it.'

'Oh, I know. That's what's done it.'

How many times do I have to learn the lesson? If I want something from a patient, if I get attached to what he or she might say to me, do for me, then it doesn't happen. After all, we are not in the treatment room in order to meet my needs. But if I can let go of what I want, if I can get back to simply attending to the patient, then it seems I am given what I need after all. I don't pretend to understand how this works, but I know that it is one of the key principles of all kinds of therapy – do the work as best you can and then let go of any desired outcome.

I saw Sean once more, about a year later. He had turned his life around. He had fallen in love with a local woman – 'It's the first time I've ever loved anyone properly and I can't believe it's happened to me, at forty-five; I didn't think I ever would, so old' – and was living happily with her. His son, from whom he had been estranged, had returned and was living with the two of them, also happily. And he had started a new business which was going well. He looked different too. Gone was his thin stick-like frame and the awkwardness of his posture; gone too the resignation of his slump in the chair. There was pink in his face instead of a greeny white.

Some things hadn't changed though. He explained that he had 'tightness' in his left leg below the knee and the physiotherapist he went to thought it must be neural and that he should have a scan. So that was booked for next week. Last month he had a rash on his neck and had been for blood, hair and urine tests from which it appeared that his mineral counts were low, and therefore there was something wrong with his Large Intestine; a leaky gut, he had been told. But he wasn't sure about the diagnosis, so he went to another doctor to be re-tested and was told that there was nothing wrong with his Large Intestine after all, and he didn't have a leaky gut, but that he did have a gluten intolerance. Oh, and he nearly forgot to tell me that his groin was always cold. There were a few more minor symptoms too.

'So what do you want from me, Sean?'

'I thought, all these separate things; they might not be separate. And what you do is you look at it all together. So I wanted to know what you think.'

'Alright.'

I checked everything. His pulses were pretty good, though they did indicate a bit of anxiety, which I hadn't picked up from what he had told me. His tongue was good too, but the tip was quite markedly red, which usually indicates some emotional distress; again it wasn't quite in line with what he had said about his new life. His structure still showed some disturbance in the energy of his left hand side which I remembered from previous treatments. But still, by comparison with how he had been, the overall picture was of improvement everywhere.

'It's all pretty good,' I said.

'Did you find anything wrong with my Large Intestine?'

'I didn't.'

'So what caused the rash, do you think?'

'No idea. You could have been overheating for some reason, or it could have been anger rising up – how is the anger, by the way?'

'It's not like it used to be. If I look for it I can find it but that's all.'

'Good.'

'So…what do you think?'

'I think that no one's body works perfectly all the time. It doesn't mean you're ill, nor that there is anything much you can do about it except the usual – eat sensibly, get enough sleep and exercise – and wait for it to pass. It may be that it is dealing with something you'll never know about, perhaps a bit of internal inflammation, or it could be a hint that you are more stressed than you realise, but again it doesn't mean there is anything wrong with you.

'I think that worrying about each and every symptom is an old habit. I am sure that you got into it, completely unconsciously, for good reasons. Maybe it was the only thing that got your mother's attention when you desperately needed it, maybe it got you off school. But it doesn't matter why you got into it. Now you are a grown man and settled with a happy family life, you don't need to go on doing it. So I suggest you just give it up.

'And although it sounds simple, it won't necessarily be easy, at least at first. All habits, like smoking or checking your emails all the time, are quite hard to give up. But there is no magic to it really. Each time you are tempted – in your case to start worrying about a symptom and going to a doctor or physiotherapist or dietician or acupuncturist – you simply don't. You don't pick up the phone and you don't start searching the internet for a diagnosis. Instead you distract yourself with some activity until you forget about it.

'The usual thoughts will pop into your mind – Why do I have this rash? Who can I go to with it? Is it a sign that something's wrong? You won't be able to help that; but what you can help is chasing the thoughts, leaping from one dire conclusion to the next, worrying about them, picking up the phone. That's the habit you have to quit.

'You're in a really good place for the first time for years, probably ever. It won't help to import into it all the old stuff from before – and this is old stuff from before. You wouldn't dream of sitting at home now, with your partner and your son, and choose to start taking drugs again. Well, don't sit at home with your partner and son and spend your time worrying about being ill.'

It was probably the longest speech I had ever given a patient. When I stopped, Sean looked at me as if to ask: is that it? I nodded. He got up. 'They aren't separate, are they?' he said. 'I thought not, but I couldn't see what they had in common. I can see now. I was looking in the wrong place.'

I smiled at that.

5

Alice's and Hugh's Depression and Reviving the Spirit

I TREAT QUITE A FEW PEOPLE FOR DEPRESSION, BUT when they first turn up to see me they hardly ever tell me that this is what ails them. A few of them don't realise they are depressed because it has come to seem normal to live with feelings of helplessness and resignation. Some are so badly affected that they say there is nothing wrong with them and they have only come because a husband or wife, an old friend or a colleague, absolutely insisted. And then there are those who don't say they are depressed because they don't like to admit it. They don't think of it like bronchitis or eczema or migraines – illnesses which happen to people but aren't their fault. Rather they see it as a weakness or failing in them to which they shouldn't have succumbed and which they should somehow be able to deal with by strength of will.

So initially people tend to give me some other reason for seeking treatment, and by far the most common is excessive tiredness. They say that they don't have the energy to play with their children, to do the sport they used to love, to go out to the cinema after work, to get up when the alarm goes off and generally participate fully in their lives. They are physically tired and they are also tired of life. Indeed, so frequent is this combination of depression and lack of energy that it has always seemed odd to me that they are regarded, at least in the West, as separate.

Roughly speaking, Western medicine has two basic approaches to depression. One is to see it as caused by an excess or deficiency of chemicals in the brain. Hence drugs are manufactured to supplement or control the naturally occurring chemicals. The other approach is to see depression as a psychological problem: as, very briefly, an inability to respond appropriately to the ups and downs of normal life. This inability will probably be found to have its roots in childhood when the patient had to invent ways of coping with unmanageable pressures or traumas. These ways, which helped at the time, then become automatic behaviours which are inappropriate in adult life. So talking therapy helps the patient to become aware of what used to be unconscious; and then he or she is free to think and act differently.

Eastern medicine has its roots in a different culture and in a different view of the body, both of which lead it to see depression as caused by a disturbance in a person's energy system. Of course it recognises that an inability to enjoy life or a mood of resignation or despair are genuine afflictions, and that things that typically leave people depressed – the death of a spouse, acute worry about money, the failure to realise one's goals or dreams in life – are hard for anyone. According to this view, what distinguishes those who come to terms with these issues from those who are overwhelmed by them is the state of the person's energy.

An analogy may help to explain the idea. When I was young there was a toy called a wibbly-wobbly man. You knocked him down and he bounced back upright. I suppose there was some kind of spring in him which gradually wore out because after a while he righted himself more and more slowly and eventually could no longer do it at all. In some people the spring, so to speak, is strong while in others it is weak – and they are the ones who find it hard to recover from being knocked down by life's misfortunes.

As a generalisation, when older people have depression it tends to be the result of a long history of disappointment and defeat; that is what has weakened the spring. With young people this weakening can happen quite quickly if they have been taking too many drugs, or have experienced a traumatic event of some kind. The consequences can range from mild to severe or even catastrophic. It is not easy to use acupuncture to treat people who are at the severe end of the spectrum. For one thing they probably need treatment every few days and this is rarely practicable, and for another they are usually on powerful anti-psychotic drugs which have such a distorting effect on the body's energy, and indeed on its whole physiology, that the signs and symptoms we normally use for diagnosis are completely unreliable.

So most of the people I treat for depression are the ones who are finding life grey and joyless, and for whom everyday basics are too much of an effort. Why get dressed, why have breakfast, why pretend any interest in what your family or friends are saying and doing? Why clean or tidy the house when it will only have to be done again tomorrow? And why bother to read a book or watch the news when nothing makes any difference?

Two new patients turned up for treatment in the same week, both of whom were in this kind of state. One was in her late teens, the other in his sixties. To my surprise I found that although they were very different in all sorts of ways, the work I needed to do was basically the same with each of them.

Alice looked bright enough when she arrived for her first treatment but she couldn't keep up appearances for long. Soon enough her voice started to trail away at the end of sentences and her gestures became slow and feeble. At first she made an effort to communicate but quite quickly her answers to my questions became short and monosyllabic. She seemed helpless, as if the stuffing had been taken out of her. It is dreadfully sad to see anyone in such a state, but somehow it is even worse when it is a young person who, by rights, should be relishing life, exploring the world and starting to find out what she wants to do in future.

A young woman of nineteen, Alice was the child of a happy marriage, with parents who could afford to give her the best of starts in life. She had done well at school, played tennis to a pretty high standard and had had a normal busy teenage social life. She wasn't at university like her friends because she had been unwell, as she put it, when she should have been taking her exams, so she had no qualifications at all. Since then she had had a series of unskilled and uninteresting jobs but she was too unreliable to keep any of them for long. On her bad days, and she told me they were frequent, it was more than she could do to leave the house and get herself to the bus stop.

I asked her what it was that stopped her and she told me about her pain. Practically every day she had a deep dragging ache low down in her abdomen, just above the pubic bone. 'It sounds like a period pain,' I said, 'but you can't have one of those every day.'

'I've got a coil,' she replied, 'so I don't have periods.'

Alarm bells were starting to ring in my head. Perhaps something had gone wrong with the coil or maybe she had endometriosis, both of which would need urgent investigation. And anyway coils don't always prevent normal periods.

I told her she absolutely had to get the coil checked out. And then I asked, 'Do you have to have it in? Could you do without it for a while and see if that's what's causing your pain?'

'I suppose so,' she agreed, though I couldn't help wondering if she had the energy to get round to doing it. I asked if she had a boyfriend – she did – and if it was an important relationship – it wasn't. She spoke of him in the same flat way she spoke about everything else.

There is sometimes a kind of anguish in the eyes of people who are in pain but Alice's were dull and lifeless as if the electricity which used to animate them had been cut off and they were only just kept going by a reserve battery which was running out of juice. It would be perfectly reasonable to think that the pain was the cause of this – after all, being in pain is terribly draining – but I didn't believe it. I thought it was more likely that it was the other way round, that somehow the pain and the deadness, which I was beginning to think was full-blown depression, were different manifestations of one condition, and that both of them sprang from one experience.

I asked her about drugs. She told me that she had smoked quite a lot of cannabis when she was at school but for the past couple of years it had only been at the weekend with friends. 'Hard drugs?' She shook her head. 'Really, no.'

If it wasn't drugs then something had happened to her, and I feared it was bad. People who have suffered from some traumatic event, who have been put in intolerable situations or undergone betrayal or abandonments, have often had to distort themselves in some way in order to survive, and that leaves its mark. With these patients, as with Alice, I often feel there is something unreal about what they tell me. It's not so much that they are covering up the reality of themselves and their lives, but that they have lost touch with it.

Later in that week I also saw Hugh for the first time. He was very clear. He told me he had post viral syndrome. He hadn't really recovered from a nasty bout of flu three months previously and he wondered if I could help.

'The main symptom?' I asked.

'Exhaustion. Weariness,' he replied. 'I'm dragging myself around.'

'Have you had it before?'

'Well, yes, but not like this.'

'What's the difference?'

'Well, this time it's not psychological. It's physical.'

'Tell me about the other times.'

Then Hugh spoke fluently of his recurrent bouts of depression. He had done this often, I realised, and it was a familiar and practised story. How his father had been killed in an accident in Africa when Hugh was nine years old; how he had returned to a cold and damp England with a grieving mother. How she had then re-married quickly – 'She didn't have much choice, poor thing, in the 1960s with four children she could barely support, working all hours.' How he didn't get on with his stepfather, so was sent away to boarding school, where he was desperately unhappy. 'After living a happy family life and running free in the sunshine of Africa it was like being thrown out of Eden.' He told me that was when he discovered his homosexuality but had to suppress it. 'It was still a criminal offence in those days. Unbelievable now.'

Although there were other bouts of depression throughout his life, Hugh traced them all back to those early experiences. He had tried many kinds of therapy which had given him insight into his depression, but they had not been able to release its hold on him.

'But I imagine you've learned how to deal with it, after all these years?'

'In a way. But I thought that because this one started with the flu I might be able to get treatment for it rather than take the tablets again and endure the long slow route back up.'

'It's true that flu can leave you feeling vey low, but I wonder if there is anything else that happened recently, something you would normally recognise as a trigger for a fresh bout of depression?'

Tears welled up in Hugh's eyes.

Finally he said, 'I'm so ashamed. I just can't forgive myself.' He seemed to be steeling himself to tell me about it.

'I don't need to know what you did.'

He shot me a grateful look.

Actually, I was grateful to him. When he said he was ashamed I suddenly thought of Alice and realised it was true for her too. It wasn't that I thought she'd done anything wrong – on the contrary, I suspected that something very wrong had been done to her – but she was ashamed of it. That was what I had missed.

When we are healthy we feel emotions but they don't linger, they come and go and we may feel half a dozen in the course of a day. But for Alice and Hugh the shame they felt did not come and go. It sat on them like a weight, squashing their natural vitality. No wonder it's called depression, I thought. When something is pressed down it can't move.

And unless you can move you can't be balanced. Our muscles work hard to keep us upright, even when standing still, let alone when we're running or riding a bicycle. Similarly, in order to stay upright emotionally we need to be reacting all the time and moving constantly back towards our centre. But when you are pressed down you cannot do that, you cannot get back up again.

Balance is fundamental. You can see it operating everywhere in the body. One group of muscles allows us to extend a limb and another group of muscles balances this movement by enabling us to flex it. We have mechanisms for preserving body heat, like hairs trapping warm air next to the skin, and balancing mechanisms for losing it, like sweating. The same happens with hormones; high levels of ACTH increases the production of hydrocortisone, which then suppresses the release of ACTH by the pituitary gland. So health is when the energies of the body are in balance; that is what keeps you well. And if you do succumb to illness then healing is the process of restoring that balance.

There are a number of ways of going about this. One is by offering patients an alternative to their attitudes and beliefs. It took a little while, but once Alice felt safe in the treatment room she did tell me what had happened to her and how it had left her feeling worthless, damaged and dirty. So I was able to explain how the body regenerates, how quickly cells die and are replaced, and how there was almost certainly not a single one of the original cells left in the places that had been affected. The idea of the conversation was to start the work of restoring some balance to her fixed view of herself.

With Hugh, who was convinced that he had done something terribly wrong and that it was irrevocable and unforgivable, it was easy to say with complete honesty (once he assured me it was not a serious crime) that everyone I knew, including myself, had done things which we wished we had not done, which we regretted deeply and for which we would always feel remorse. He was no different from the rest of us. Or, more accurately, the only difference was that we had somehow managed to get over our cruelties and failures, while he had not. I was hoping to provide some sense of balance to his resignation.

Hugh was a tall man but he looked as if he had caved in. His head fell forward, his chest was sunken and his voice was very quiet, all of which spoke eloquently of a weakness in the energy of his lungs. In all traditional medicines that speaks of grief and of an inability to be inspired by life.

> In a balanced body inspiration involves lengthening of the entire spine, from the sacrum all the way up to the cranium. When movements are restricted, individuals can no longer feel an emotion as an emotion. No longer can they have a natural response to an immediate situation and then get on with their life. (Oschman 2000, p.161)

This described Hugh very well and it made me realise that he probably didn't even know he was in grief. At some stage, I thought, I should warn him that he might have to feel it afresh as part of his recovery.

Grief is always linked to the lungs. It isn't hard to see why. The violent spasms of the lungs produce the typical sobbing and wailing of grief, and weaken them. So Hugh's treatment was directed towards re-energising his lungs. As the weeks went by, the front of his body started to open out, uncoiling him and making space for something new to enter his life, helping him, in the words of the quotation above, to have a 'natural response to an immediate situation'.

Then one day he told me he had bought a notebook – he called it his atonement book. In it he was writing exactly what he had done that he was so ashamed of, sparing no detail. It was his way of saying he was sorry. If he couldn't say it to those he believed he had harmed then at least he could own up to it in writing.

'What will you do with the book once you've finished it?'

'I hadn't thought. Why do you ask?'

'Well, I think it is a great idea, but I am not sure about keeping it on your bookshelf once you've finished it.'

'You think I should throw it away?'

'Oh, I think it deserves more than that. You could have a bonfire.'

'And dance around it as it burned?' Hugh laughed.

That was the first time I ever heard him laugh and I will always remember it. It was such a good sign. Shakespeare, as so often, puts his finger on it – 'present mirth hath present laughter' (Twelfth Night, Act II, Scene III, line 47). In other words Hugh was in the present at last, instead of the past.

It was helpful that I was treating Hugh and Alice concurrently, as the thoughts and ideas I had about one of them illuminated what I needed to do with the other. When I became aware of the stagnation of energy in Hugh's lungs it made me wonder if the same might be true of Alice's lower abdomen. I asked her to feel all three areas of her torso when she woke up in the morning – upper chest, rib cage to umbilicus, and lower abdomen – to see if they were the same temperature. She reported that the lower one was colder. I asked if I could feel it and indeed it was strikingly cold to the touch and it felt lifeless too.

That led me to a specific treatment for cold in the uterus. It also gave me the opportunity to explain how when we are hurt somewhere then, all unconsciously, we sometimes withdraw our energy from that area of the body. It's a way of protecting ourselves from unbearable feelings – which is helpful at the time, but in the long run it means that area won't have the energy it needs to change and to heal. The treatment I was going to do would bring energy back into her lower abdomen.

'Does that mean I'll have to experience it all over again?'

It was a fair question. I had to be honest.

'I don't know. It might. But if it does you will know it is in a safe place, you'll know that this time it is healing rather than damaging, and that this time it will pass.'

Bravely, she agreed.

From that time on the pain started to subside. She did eventually have the coil out and was better for it, though I did end up thinking it wasn't the main cause. And as the pain ebbed away what was left was a young woman who could function again. She got a job as a receptionist in a small company with people she liked and who respected her. She arranged to go travelling with a friend in the summer, which I saw as the beginning of catching up with what she should have been doing in those lost years.

Alice was very much better in all sorts of ways but her spirits were still low. We all know perfectly well what that means and we all know what it looks like too. There is no lift in the voice, no sparkle in the eyes, no quick and ready smile, and the person seems a tiny bit like an automaton, going through the motions of normal life. It is also a well-understood diagnosis in Chinese medicine, though not in the West. There are plenty of acupuncture points which treat the patient's spirit generally, and some which have very specific effects. The point called Spirit Storehouse, for example, replenishes spirits which have become depleted and exhausted; the one called Spirit Seal, on the other hand, is more an affirmation of an individual's unique identity. I remembered that my very first impression of Alice was that she didn't know who she was.

In what I hoped would be Alice's last few treatments I used spirit points like these. I had the image that the previous treatments had been building a house – laying foundations, putting the roof on, connecting the services and so on, but until I did these points the place was empty and no one was living there. And it worked. After that she came back once more, a few months later for a treatment after her beloved grandfather's death, which she had found hard. Although she was sad, of course, it was a joy to see her looking so well.

And these last few treatments with her helped me to see Hugh afresh. He wasn't nearly as depressed as he had been but he had got stuck somewhere on the road to recovery. I was now seeing him every three weeks and it was as if each treatment picked him up but then he would fall over again and couldn't get back on his feet by himself. I felt we weren't making progress.

So now it wasn't just that Hugh was stuck, I was too. For me, one of the most frustrating things about being a practitioner is when a patient does very well at first but then the improvement stops and won't budge. Almost always it is because I am missing something and I just can't see what it is. It usually takes something unforeseen to jolt me out of my tunnel vision, and this time it was the happenstance that Hugh's appointment one day came straight after Alice's.

I was about to needle the first point on Hugh when I suddenly realised I was in the wrong place. My attention must have lapsed because I found myself about to needle the last point I had done on Alice instead of the one I was planning to do on Hugh. When I was a novice I would have tutted at myself for being so inattentive and gone immediately to the point I had planned to do, but from long experience I have come to value these mistakes. They are often gifts we are given when we manage to stop thinking for a moment, gifts that come from our unconscious knowledge and experience.

Sometimes, of course, mistakes really are mistakes, so I did pause to reflect before going ahead and needling Alice's spirit point, as I called it. But I liked the idea of using it on Hugh. For one thing, it was a new approach, and I sorely needed that. And for another it would take treatment to a different level. I had done all sorts of treatments, but I hadn't treated his spirit. I allowed myself a silent shake of the head. It was so obvious I couldn't imagine why I hadn't thought of it before – still can't, as a matter of fact. It was like one of those annoying card games where the one you need is right in front of you but somehow you can't see it until it's too late.

Luckily it wasn't too late and from then on Hugh improved steadily. It made me think of those remarkable Chinese acupuncturists, not centuries ago but millennia ago, who found out that specific points could treat the spirit in specific ways. How did they know? What were their methods? And I couldn't help thinking what powerful intellects they must have had to bring all their knowledge together into a coherent system.

And here we were, Alice, Hugh and me, the beneficiaries of all their work, finding out that what they discovered is still true and still helping people who live in a culture, in a society, and in a technological world which would have been utterly unimaginable to them. I find it very reassuring that such wisdom persists.

6

Pauline's Headaches and Treating the Patient

HEADACHES COME IN A HUNDRED DIFFERENT shapes and sizes, maybe more. The pain can be sharp and intense, fixed and throbbing, dull and achy, like a tight hat or an iron vice. The head may feel full to bursting with cotton wool or as if it is holding a bag of coins which rattle around and bang against the inside of the skull. It can be worse in the morning, the evening, on waking, just before a period, or at random intervals. The pain can be on one of the temples, on both, on the forehead, the back or top of the head, deep inside, just behind the eyes or a combination of some, or many, of the above. Quite a few are accompanied by nausea or disturbed vision – indeed the eyes can be so badly affected that the sufferer has to stay in a darkened room until they pass. Sitting upright may take the edge off one person's headache while lying down may relieve another's. A firm massage on the skull may feel great or terrible. And so on.

So the starting point with any headache is to accept straight away that what works for one person may not work for anyone else; and that where a patient has more than one kind of headache, which is not unusual, what helps one of their headaches might not help with the others.

All of which presents any medical practitioner with a fundamental challenge. The basic procedure of all medicine is to look at the patient's signs and symptoms and then fit them into one of the well-known categories of illness or disease. The Western doctor who comes to the conclusion that her patient's headache is caused by meningitis or intracranial pressure, for example, is using exactly the same kind of reasoning as an acupuncturist diagnosing Kidney Yin deficiency leading to Liver Yang rising. They are both seeing in their patient an instance of something which they and others have seen before, and so will treat as they have treated before. But although it would be ridiculous to ignore all the learning and experience which is summed up in the generalisations of the medical textbooks, still, both doctor and acupuncturist are uncomfortably aware that their generalisations won't necessarily apply to the particular headache of the particular patient in front of them.

The solution to this dilemma has been pointed out by many wise doctors over the centuries, but Sir William Osler said it as well as anyone: 'The good physician treats the disease; the great physician treats the patient who has the disease' (Osler, cited in Adams 1999, p.67). In other words the treatment, however deeply rooted in the classifications of theory and practice, has to be crafted anew for each patient.

It isn't always easy to do so, and many practitioners, especially when short of time and under pressure of work, tend to ignore this truth and fall back on treating the disease, hoping to offer symptomatic relief. When this works it is tempting to decide that nothing else is necessary or possible, but every now and then a patient turns up who presents the challenge in so stark a form that it simply cannot be ignored. Enter Pauline.

And when I say enter, I mean enter. Pauline does not slip unnoticed into a room. Somewhat like a ship on the high seas – no, make that a galleon – she moves ahead with a big bow wave and a sense of unstoppable force. Not that she is tall; it is entirely the power of her personality. I am sure she has always had a presence, but at the age of sixty, it comes with the additional power of a person who is well known and hugely respected in her profession.

Twenty years ago she was the owner and manager of a well-known restaurant in the West End of London, and from what she told me she must have run it with a combination of panache and iron discipline. But one day, all those years ago, and apparently out of the blue – though, looking back on it, she came to see it as the culmination of many years of stress at work – she collapsed. And the headaches started. For the next year she hardly left her bed and doubted that she would ever get better. Doctors of all sorts prescribed medicines and procedures of every kind but none of them touched the headaches. After that she was never well enough to run the restaurant again and she had to sell it – 'it was like losing an arm' she told me. Some years later she became a food critic and writer and she travels endlessly, seeking out and describing foods of every nation and culture. What she writes is always both expert and fair, so she is welcomed by restauranteurs the world over.

Whatever the time of her treatment Pauline is always dressed as if for a smart occasion: skirt and jacket, silk blouse and necklace, full make-up and long blonde hair carefully coiled on the top of her head. And, although it is slightly surprising in one so impeccably presented, she carries with her a natural and generous warmth. There is absolutely no doubt that Pauline is the staunchest of friends and the kindest of neighbours, though if you catch the sharp appraising look in her eye, you will know that she does not suffer fools gladly.

The first time she walked into my treatment room she looked around carefully, nodded approvingly and then told me she had headaches. And I said to myself, as if I didn't know better – Well,

I should be able to help alright; acupuncture is really good for headaches. I hadn't reckoned with Pauline's headaches.

It turned out she had three kinds. The first, which she has whenever she doesn't have one of the others, is a thick, dense, fuzzy feeling which takes over the whole of the inside of her head and leaves it numb on top. She said she doesn't mind it too much as she can function when she has it.

She calls the second kind of headache a migraine, though it differs in a number of ways from what are usually called migraines. For one thing the pain is on her forehead whereas a typical migraine is usually on one of the temples; and for another, her migraines don't come with either nausea or visual disturbance. Still, for some reason, the medication she was given for migraines works for these headaches, and if she takes a pill as soon as they start then the pain eases off within an hour or two.

But when the pill doesn't work she knows she is about to get the third kind of headache, which she calls a tsunami headache. The pain fills her whole head, lasts for three or four days and is severe and relentless. Nothing alleviates a tsunami headache, not even really powerful painkillers, and there is nothing she can do to get it over with quickly. And all the while she is completely and utterly incapacitated. Finally, after a few days and for no apparent reason, it simply clears by itself. As far as I can tell, a tsunami headache is unknown to Eastern medicine as it is to Western.

It didn't seem sensible to try and diagnose each kind of headache separately and then treat it separately, so I chose a systemic treatment. In any case the only headache for which I could come up with a convincing diagnosis was the first kind, the background headache, and that was the only one she could live with.

So I did a treatment which clears what are called 'lingering pathogens'. The basic idea of this treatment is best summed up by an experience I had with a car I once owned. It was fast and it was wonderful to drive but only rarely would it start in the morning. A common sight in the village where I lived, and one which amused the neighbours greatly, was me pushing it down the street to try and get the engine to engage. The garage never managed to fix it, so one day I took it to a specialist mechanic who kept it for well over a week. When I collected it he assured me that it would start now, and indeed I never had the slightest problem with it afterwards. 'What was it?' I asked. 'No one else has been able to find what was wrong with it.' 'No idea,' he replied cheerfully. 'I took everything out, cleaned it, and put it all back again, and it seems to have done the trick.'

Given that Pauline had been unwell for the best part of twenty years and that no one had ever identified a cause of her headaches, this seemed to be the right kind of treatment to start with.

A week later she told me she thought I was on the right lines. 'Only the background headache this week – but then I might not have had one of the others. It's just that I've been better in myself.' That last sentence is one of my favourite things to hear from any patient, better even than a clear improvement in any symptom. For it points to a body beginning to recover its natural ability to restore health.

Although I still didn't have anything like a diagnosis of Pauline's various headaches, I did have some pointers as to what was going on and they indicated two well-known kinds of treatment: one to relieve stagnation of blood and the other to clear phlegm; so that's what I did. Pauline reported that although she continued to get the first two kinds of headaches they were less frequent and less severe than before.

And then one day she rang me to say she had a full-blown tsunami headache. Her husband brought her to me – she couldn't have driven herself. I wanted to see if a treatment could make any difference to a tsunami headache, and in any case it was a golden opportunity to get good feedback.

Her pulses would give me the first kind of feedback. In my experience a patient's pulses give a completely reliable readout of the effects of treatment. That is, if the pulses don't change at all after I have put the needles in, it either means that I have missed the point or that those points were irrelevant to the patient's condition. I take the needles out and think again. Another possibility is that the pulses all get worse; those that were tight become tighter, those that were weak become weaker and so on. That is an unequivocal message that what I am doing is aggravating the patient's condition. Again, I take the needles out and think again, but this time with a more precise and powerful indication of what is needed – normally exactly the opposite of what I have done. The last possibility is that all the pulses improve markedly. That is, if they were weak and slow they become stronger and faster; if they were pushy and fast then they become calmer and slow down – there are endless varieties of change for the better, but all of them indicate that the treatment is working and that the patient's energy is moving back into balance.

And treating Pauline while in the grip of a tsunami meant that I would also be able to get additional feedback, as she would be able to report whether or not the points I was using were alleviating the pain. That would give me an invaluable comparison. For if I thought, from the pulses, that the headache was easing and Pauline said the same, then I would know that I could trust my reading of her pulses in future. And, of course, if I was wrong I could start to work out what I had missed or misunderstood.

So I was in a cheerful mood when I put the needles in. All went according to plan. Her pulses, which had been initially hard, fast and sharp – as if they were attacking my fingertips – started to slow down and soften. The colour of her face which had been a blotchy mixture of vivid reds and yellows faded to a healthier-looking pink. And best of all, she reported that the pain was shrinking and easing too.

I monitored progress by taking her pulses repeatedly and also asking her for regular reports, until by the end of about half an hour, the pain was reduced to a small and mild ache and the pulses had gone back to what they were like when she didn't have a headache. I left the needles in a minute or two longer, 'just to be on the safe side' as I say to myself, even though I know it doesn't really make any sense at all; either the needles have finished their work or they haven't. Then I took them out and, something I learned many years ago from one of my teachers, I re-checked the pulses one last time to make sure that all was well before saying that the treatment was finished.

But all was not well. Within moments the pulses started to go hard, like quick-drying cement, and by the time I got to the last one they were all more or less back to where they had been when I first checked them. And as I put Pauline's hand down I glanced at her face and I knew, seconds before she told me, that her headache was back in full force.

This was new for me. Certainly, in the past, I have taken needles out and found that one or two of the patient's pulses have got a bit worse, showing me that I have overlooked something that needed attention, or that there was a bit more to do before finishing the treatment, but never before had I been given an unequivocal message that the treatment had made no difference at all, that I might as well have done nothing.

What to do? It wasn't a matter of fine tuning a treatment or adding a finishing touch, as in the past. This was new. So I did what I had never done before, and haven't done since, simply because I couldn't think of anything else to do. I got some new needles and put them all in exactly the same places as all the old ones.

Another half an hour and everything seemed to have settled down, but as I expect you will have guessed, when I took those needles out the same thing happened again. So I did the same again. I'd like to say that I had a theory, that I had good reason to believe that this was one of those cases where the needles had to be in not for the customary twenty minutes or so but for sixty or more, but it wouldn't be true. I just didn't have a better idea. And Pauline, thankfully, was willing to let me try. 'It's not as if anything else has ever worked,' she said.

One of the wonderful, and terrifying, things about being an acupuncturist is that, rather like a musician or an actor on stage, the work has to be done there and then, however nervous you are and however inadequate you feel. You don't have much time to think, nor can you wait until the patient has had a barrage of tests before you commit yourself to a treatment. You are faced with hard questions which demand immediate answers; do you do something that is well known and understood, for example, even if it seems not to be working; or do you try something new and take the risk that it may make things worse? And often enough, as with Pauline, there is the added pressure that acupuncture is the patient's last hope.

Luckily, the third time I did the identical treatment it worked. That time the pulses stayed slow and soft even after the needles were out, and the pain didn't come back. 'It fought back,' said Pauline. 'But so did we.'

It was a kind thing to say. It didn't criticise me for failing to disperse the headache at the first or even the second attempt and it freed me of the burden of being some kind of heroic figure who is supposed to fix whatever problem the patient brings to me, a role which I find both uncomfortable and unrealistic.

After that enormous session things improved quite a bit. The tsunami headache seemed to acknowledge the strength and persistence of its adversary, and in future treatments it would ease with only one round of needles. She still had all three kinds of headaches but she had them less often and they were less severe. From now on, I thought, it would be a matter of small incremental changes until, sooner or later, her headaches would become occasional irritants rather than frequent severe pains.

But that's not what happened, and after another six months of treatment there was no further improvement. I knew there were good reasons for persisting. For one thing, her headaches might get worse again if she stopped. And then, perhaps, and for some unaccountable reason, one day a single treatment might make all the difference. I thought of a steel bar which can weaken imperceptibly over many years, but then breaks in a moment. Perhaps the cumulative effects of all Pauline's treatments were indeed wearing away at the stuckness of her condition, and it simply needed persistence on both our parts for the headaches to fade away. I acknowledged these possibilities, but the truth was I had run out of ideas and I was losing heart.

Finally I sat down and really took stock of all my time and treatments with Pauline and I thought of the quotation I referred to earlier: 'The good physician treats the disease; the great physician treats the patient who has the disease.' And I realised that I hadn't actually been a great physician. On the contrary, I had seen her headaches as alien things which weren't really part of her, like ivy growing up a tree, and I thought I could simply remove them. And, of course, that meant that I had not been treating her. So who was she, before and behind those headaches? Underneath that immaculate front she presented to the world? I asked myself these questions repeatedly over the next year and I was endlessly frustrated by my inability to answer them.

A glimmer of light did come when I was mulling over the fact that she used an image of unstoppable water energy, a tsunami, to describe her really bad headaches. So, along the same lines, I thought that a migraine might be like a flood and a background headache like a trickle. Perhaps they were all the effects of water energy. But why would water energy give her headaches? I supposed that if water was flowing into a container that was too small, like over-filling a bag or balloon, then it might put an enormous strain on that container – in this instance the skull. But water didn't flow upwards, so how could it get to her head? It didn't make sense – unless, that is, the water was boiling. And then I realised, in one of those rare moments when the obvious comes into view, that boiling water both rises and expands. That would do it, I thought; that would put pressure on the meninges of the skull.

I was still a long way from a proper understanding of Pauline's headaches; for one thing I had no idea why her body fluids might be boiling, and although there were some signs of heat on her pulses and tongue, it didn't seem severe. Still, in her unforgettable words, nothing else had worked, so I needled all the cooling points I could think of and added points which would pull rising energy downwards.

I thought of James Watt watching the tight lid of a kettle being pushed up by boiling water; and I remembered my mother's pressure cooker which had to be made of very thick steel so it didn't explode. I asked myself, What other kind of energy has this sense of contained pressure? and the answer that came back was the energy of frustration. I thought of how with frustration, the mouth goes tight and the fists clench and there is an intensity of feeling inside which is not vented. So I wondered for the first time if Pauline was constantly frustrated by having to write about restaurants when she really wanted to be running them. I could imagine how every time she was in a restaurant she admired, or maybe even more in one which she thought she could improve, she must long to roll her sleeves up and take over.

When Pauline turned up the next time there was a change in her. The only way I can describe it is to say that she seemed less tight. Her clothes looked floppier on her, her glance was less sharp, and her footfall, which previously made me think of marching jackboots, was quieter.

So I started to treat her frustration rather than her headaches, and it really was like slowly opening that little valve on the top of a pressure cooker. Over the next few months her body seemed to relax a little, her eyes became softer, and she started to lose that rather fearsome air she carried about with her. There was not much change in her headaches and I did wonder occasionally if I was doing right; but I consoled myself with the thought that I couldn't bring about this kind of relaxation with my needles unless there was a part of her that was willing to allow it. Unconsciously, did she want to let go a bit, to take life more easily and stop yearning to be back in charge?

My treatments were better than they had been but all I was doing, really, was dispersing some of her pent-up frustration. Instead of stopping a dripping tap I was just emptying the bath when it got too full. The usual view is that the kind of treatment that finally stops the dripping tap comes when the practitioner has reached the correct diagnosis – and indeed I might not have done so. But in my experience it more often comes when something happens in the treatment room which seems to draw away a veil which has kept me from seeing the reality of the person and his or her ailment. It can happen when the patient and I have had a conversation which is somehow deeper and more resonant than usual, when we gain some new insight and explore it together. Or it can happen in the moment a needle touches a point, when we both relax into the new energetic state that has been created and let out a sigh of relief as we do so. Or it can come, as it did with a patient recently, when she suddenly saw that the disability which she had tried to hide from the world was actually a badge of honour, the living proof of her bravery.

It is different every time, but what all instances have in common is that afterwards I feel I know the patient in a way I haven't before and we both know we are in new territory together. But to my regret it hasn't happened with Pauline.

It's been nearly four years now and she still comes for treatment regularly. The background headaches are milder, the migraines are less frequent, and at the time of writing this she hasn't had a tsunami for four months, which is definitely a record. So there has been an improvement but I still wish I had been able to do more. At one time I suggested she go to another practitioner, one I know well and respect; perhaps he would see something I had missed, think of a diagnosis I had overlooked, or be able to see her more clearly than I had managed to do. But Pauline refused. 'I'm not starting all over again. And anyway,' she smiled, 'he might be worse than you.'

Shortly before writing this she arrived with an announcement. 'I've started to meditate,' she said. 'It's brilliant, really helping.'

I was astonished, and it must have shown.

'Don't look at me like that,' she said. 'I like it. Why didn't you tell me to all those years ago?'

'I thought you wouldn't take me seriously if I did. I thought you'd never come back.'

'You're right, I wouldn't have done.'

It might be that taking up meditation will cure her headaches, but if it isn't that I think it will be something else. For Pauline has courage and is willing to look at what is difficult or uncomfortable in her life, so I do believe that one day, sooner or later, she will realise what has to be done in order to be rid of them. And then she will undertake whatever it requires of her and her life. And the part acupuncture will have played? It didn't cure her headaches, but perhaps it will have opened up the possibility of change.

Reflections on Sean, Alice, Hugh and Pauline

All of these patients had very difficult experiences in their lives and none of them had managed to fully recover. They weren't ill in the sense of having a disease, but they were ill in the sense of having chronic pain or long-term problems. Although practically nothing is known about the way that difficult experiences manifest in the body and become physical symptoms, every practitioner has seen this so often in their patients that it is impossible to doubt. There has been some scientific research (Hunt 1989; Pert 1997), which suggests that emotional stress changes a person's energy and that tissue change then follows. If that is the case then perhaps acupuncture, and other forms of complementary medicine, restore health by restoring the patient's original energy.

With these patients I couldn't know what their original energy was like, but by the time I saw them it was constrained, tight, held in and repressed. For good reasons, Sean had buried his anger deep; Alice and Hugh had hidden their sense of shame; and Pauline had stifled her real ambition. Accordingly, I came to see Sean's multiple symptoms as a host of tiny shoots of growth, like plants coming up round the edges of a concrete driveway, while Alice and Hugh's depression was more like an enormous weight of unbearable thoughts and memories. And Pauline's headaches seemed to come from a brain bursting with plans and ideas which she was powerless to implement.

The first goal of treatment, then, was to mitigate the pressure they were under. Sean responded well to treatments that were comforting, reassuring and supportive; they seemed to reach a part of him that had been untouched for a long time and that gave him the confidence to open up about the bullying he had endured. Hugh and Alice both had a powerful inner critic, and for each of them it seems to have crushed their spirits and their powers of recovery alike.

And they also needed a new perspective on their illnesses. It took Sean some time to take proper account of his anger, but when he did he was then able to rail at what had happened to him as a child and let go of at least some of the distress it had caused him. Alice needed to know that her body was not permanently tainted by what had happened to her and Hugh to see that whatever he had done it was not unforgivable. Before working with these patients I hadn't really appreciated how this combination of a new energetic state and a new perspective on an illness might have considerably more power than either of them alone.

But none of this applied to Pauline. I couldn't find a treatment which revived some kind of original energy in her, nor could I come up with a sufficiently new perspective on her headaches. It is true that treatments which dispersed the energy rising to her head did alleviate the pain and the duration of her tsunami headaches, but I was never able to treat the root cause because I never found it. And it is also true that while I showed her the part that frustration had played in her headaches, it was more a trigger than a cause. As always, our failures teach us more than our successes.

And the contrast between Pauline on the one hand and Sean, Alice and Hugh on the other showed me something else as well.

There were moments with the latter three when something happened which was not a matter of diagnosis in the conventional sense, but which nevertheless turned out to be crucial. With Sean it was the sudden insight that the anger I was feeling was really his. With Alice it was remembering what Hugh had said about shame and realising it was true for her too. And with Hugh it was the mistake of starting to needle the point I had just done on Alice. These were turning points in their treatments. They somehow opened the door to a deeper level of work and to sessions which yielded more change than I had managed with normal diagnoses and procedures. For some reason, there were no such moments with Pauline.

This led me to think about exactly what an acupuncturist is doing in a treatment, and hence how it affects a patient. The normal view of it is that the practitioner has learned a theory which explains the causes of illness and disease and then applies that theory to the patient. The better the fit the more effective the treatment. But this isn't really what happened with these patients. Although I started with the familiar categories of energy disturbance and distortion, none of them really applied. Instead I was feeling my way, learning more and more about these people, both from talking to them and from seeing the results of each treatment. It wouldn't be unfair to say that I didn't know what I was doing – until, that is, I did know what I was doing. This process is somewhat like an art or a craft. A potter tries a new shape or a new glaze and finds it isn't quite right, so she changes it a bit and tries again. A pianist practising a sonata for the first time experiments with different ways of playing a passage until he is satisfied that it is both right in itself and fits well with the rest of the piece. It is a bit like that.

I think that this kind of exploration and learning through treatment is much more common in the experience of acupuncture than is normally recognised. It is as if acupuncturists operate with two distinct theories. One is the theory they were taught at college, a theory they learned well and which sits in the background, informing everything they do. And the other theory is the one they use every day when faced with a huge variety of patients, a huge variety of conditions and a very limited amount of time to think. This theory is the outcome of years of experience and habit, and it is highly individual: a mixture of rules of thumb, favourite points, reliance on a few familiar diagnostic categories, some hunches, and a style of working which owes much to the acupuncturist's particular personality.

Using this second theory allows the practitioner to adapt the work to suit each individual patient. For example, I used to have a habit of explaining, at least in general terms, what I was doing in a treatment and why I was doing it – until one day a patient lifted his head from the couch and said, in a kindly tone of voice, 'Do you think I could have the treatment without the lecture, please?' Since then I have been very aware of the need to modify the way I practise in order to find a good match between what suits me and what suits the patient.

I think this process of matching is crucial because it determines the nature of the relationship between patient and practitioner. If I come across as an expert who can work out what has gone wrong and put it right, then that takes all responsibility off the patient. It can feel reassuring, of course, but I think it is deeply misleading because treatment, however powerful and helpful, can only be a small part of a patient's life. He or she will need to play a part too. If, on the other hand, patient and practitioner can come to some kind of mutual understanding of what has happened and what needs to be done to put it right, then they will be working as partners. Then they can work more quickly, they can go deeper, and the patient will naturally begin to take on what has to be done outside the treatment room in order to be well again.

Looking back at these four patients, this kind of collaboration meant that Sean was willing to investigate his anger, that Alice could manage to tell me what had happened to her, and that Hugh could write his atonement book. I don't think any of these things would have happened unless we had come to see the process of treatment as a joint undertaking, with each of us contributing what we could. And what these patients managed to do also served to show me 'the patient who has the disease' – the person I really needed to treat. To my regret, I don't think I have ever treated that person in Pauline.

7

Anna's Miscarriages and the Power of Commitment

I'VE NEVER EXPERIENCED MOST OF THE CONDITIONS which my patients bring to me. I suppose it doesn't matter that I don't know what it feels like to have a migraine or an irritable bowel, for example, as plenty of patients with conditions like these do well with acupuncture, so I set about treating them without giving it a second thought. In theory it is just the same with gynaecological problems, but it doesn't feel like that. Because I can't ever know what it is like to have painful periods, a difficult pregnancy or a miscarriage, I feel as if I am not really entitled to speak about them; so I am always grateful when a woman is completely natural and at ease as she tells me intimate details about her body and the way it behaves.

And right from the start Anna was direct and to the point. A tall woman of thirty-eight, the chief executive of an American company which imported beauty products into the UK and every inch a professional, she talked in sentences that were so clear and concise that it was almost as if she had drafted them and revised them before speaking.

She and her husband both badly wanted children. She had no trouble becoming pregnant, but in the past fifteen months she had miscarried three times. One pregnancy had lasted four weeks, another ten weeks, and the last, most heartbreakingly of all, three and a half months. It was devastating. To have what you wanted so much, to be celebrating inside, if not publicly, and then to have it snatched away from you, not once but three times in a row – well, I couldn't imagine how she had managed to hold it all together, to keep working, and to keep on presenting herself so immaculately to the world. By sheer willpower, I guessed, which can carry people through the most enormous adversity, though normally at a price.

So what was happening? As you would expect, Anna had seen four consultants, had taken every test imaginable and she had ended up with no more idea of what was causing the miscarriages than at the start. She was coming to me with an open mind but not much more. She found it hard to believe that acupuncture could somehow do the miraculous but she was willing to give it a go. She was as frank about this as about everything else.

She told me about her periods, and I'd never heard anything quite like them. They were regular to the day every four weeks – and to the hour as well. That would normally lead me to think that she was in good health and that the extraordinarily complex and interrelated sub systems which govern menstruation were all working properly. On the other hand the bleeding went on for seven days and for the middle three days the flow was, in her own words, 'ridiculously heavy and uncontrollable'. So all was not well after all. And I pricked up my ears at the word 'uncontrollable'; did anyone ever think her menstrual flow might be controlled? Finally her blood was very dark red, which usually means there is some stagnation somewhere – but how could there be stagnation if she bled so heavily? Plenty to ponder.

I started to ask all the usual questions and she immediately told me that she had a history of eating disorders. It was as if she wanted to own up to it straight away and to have it out in the open. From the ages of thirteen to seventeen, she said, she had been seriously bulimic.

'Those teenage years can be difficult,' I commented. But she was not interested in going back into the past, nor in my rather clumsy offer of sympathy.

'I'm not over it,' she said. 'You'd think I would be, after twenty years, but I'm not.'

'How bad is it?' I asked.

As soon as I said it I wished I hadn't used the word 'bad'; it can so easily be heard as judgemental. 'Severe' or 'acute' would have been better, or even the entirely neutral 'Tell me about it.'

But Anna swept past it without a moment's hesitation. 'I don't make myself sick anymore but I binge and then starve myself; I either cut out sugar or I eat too much of it and get terrific rushes; and sometimes I snack all day and don't have a proper meal at all. In fact I hardly ever have a proper meal.'

I looked at her tongue. It was distinctly pale and had the scalloped edges which are caused by it being a little swollen and therefore pushing against the teeth at each side, like an obese person in an economy-class seat on a plane. A big tongue speaks of fluids stagnating rather than flowing, and of a weakness of the spleen which is responsible for putting the right amount of everything in its right place. The pale colour usually means that the blood is deficient or that there is a lack of Yang energy, the kind that powers a person through the day. So the overall picture was one of deficiency, of weakness and of depletion. But that was in dramatic contrast to her powerful and forthright manner. What was going on?

Making a full diagnosis entails putting together information from a wide range of sources – lots of pieces have to be put in place before the picture on the jigsaw puzzle becomes clear. No doubt all acupuncturists have different ways of assembling all these different bits of information, but my habit is to keep a running check on my thoughts and ideas. After looking at Anna's tongue, for example, I made a mental note that I expected her pulses to be deep and weak – I assumed there wouldn't be enough energy to lift them up forcefully to my fingers on the radial artery. So if, when I came to take the pulses, I found that they were strong and pushy, I would know that my initial idea was wrong.

Another way of keeping a running check on myself is to ask a question or two based on the first piece of information alone – in this instance on the state of her tongue. So I asked if she took any exercise, or did she find it too tiring?

'I run a ridiculous amount.' She seemed to be fond of the word 'ridiculous'. 'At least thirty-five miles a week. And not on roads – it's fell running.' In other words on the rough paths which criss-cross the steep hills around the village where she lives.

'Even on weekdays?' I couldn't keep the surprise out of my voice. 'How do you find the time?'

'I leave the house at seven in the morning.'

'In winter? When it's dark? When it's raining?'

'Usually, yes. I don't mind. I like it.'

Well, my first assumption was indeed wrong – she must have enough energy after all. Still, maybe she was forcing her system to do more than it really could, and the running could be depleting her. So I asked if she worked long hours. It turned out she commuted for half an hour each way and rarely got home much before seven at night.

'And then you cook? Or does your husband do the cooking?'

'No. We eat cold food. He has a hot meal at lunchtime, at work.'

'And you?'

'No. I eat cold food all the time.'

I could hardly wait to take her pulses but I decided to get one more piece of information first. I asked if I could put my hand on her belly, both above and below the umbilicus. She agreed and pulled up her blouse in the matter-of-fact way I was now coming to expect of her. The belly was a little cold to the touch above the umbilicus, but below it was really cold. Things were beginning to make sense. Cold food, a cold uterus, and lifestyle of over-exertion; not an ideal environment for a growing fetus.

And at last I took her pulses. They were indeed very deep and weak and they were slow as well, yet another sign that there was cold in the body. Two of the pulses were so weak I could barely feel them at all, the pericardium and three heater, which, briefly, govern circulation and temperature control. So her body was doing its best to keep her circulation going and to keep her base temperature at the level that the organs need, but it seemed that the effort was draining her.

So the first goals of treatment were obvious – to eliminate the cold in her body and then to strengthen her blood; plenty to be going on with. And I was very aware that she was thirty-eight years old so I would need to recruit her to the cause, otherwise progress would be too slow. She would need to change her diet and she would have to start having hot meals regularly. For someone with a history of eating disorders this might be quite a challenge. And then I thought that she should cut down on the running, at least on cold mornings, and that would be another challenge too. But far from being an obstacle I thought these challenges might be a spur to change.

For one thing I was pretty sure that Anna would rise to any challenge, and for another it would lead her away from thinking that if only she could find the right treatment her problem would be solved. This, it seemed to me, was her underlying assumption, one she had never really noticed let alone questioned, and I thought it would be good to switch her attention away from finding someone who could identify a specific malfunction of her womb or reproductive system and focus it instead on the power she had to amplify her own health.

So I said that getting warm and building up her blood were both necessary, though they might not be sufficient. Once that had been done we might find there was more to do, but unless they were done I didn't believe anything else would work. As I spoke I could see Anna thinking about it, could see her taking the idea on board, and a look of interest crossed her face. It was enough to encourage me to give her one more thing to do. It was something which looks a bit peculiar at first sight, so I was waiting to see how she responded to the other ideas before suggesting it.

There is a very ancient treatment in Chinese medicine which involves burning a herb called moxa. Sometimes it is formed into a cone and then placed on an acupuncture point and set alight so that it sends both heat and the essence of the herb down into the point (it is taken off before it burns the skin). Alternatively, and this was my idea for Anna, it comes in the form of a stick about six inches long and the thickness of a thumb. The end of the stick is lit and is then waved above the skin, gently warming an area of the body. It is a wonderful treatment for a woman soon after childbirth when the abdomen has so suddenly become cold and empty. Well, Anna's abdomen was cold and empty too. I explained why I thought it would help and exactly how she could do it herself, every day for a week. She looked a bit doubtful but agreed to give it a go.

After all that I gave her a treatment, a very simple one. I wanted to know how her body would respond to the needles and to a change in its temperature regulation. The simpler the treatment the clearer the feedback it provides.

When she had gone I sat in my treatment room and reflected that it had been a very big session for Anna. Arriving with no expectations, except perhaps that she would be covered with needles, there had been a lot of talking which ended with a new perspective on a crucial issue. And on top of that she had committed herself to a radical change in her habits, and even to waving a burning stick over her belly. I couldn't help wondering if I had gone too far and demanded too much. And I had done so before I had even started to get to know she would respond to me and to my needles.

And I reflected that it had been a big session for me too. Of course I want all my patients to get better, but this was especially important. If the treatment worked it would change Anna's and her husband's lives for ever; and if it didn't, where could she go next? What's more, if it didn't work she would have wasted time seeing me – and she couldn't afford to waste time. So I knew that treatment would be a challenge for both of us.

Her feedback from the first three or four treatments, and from using the moxa stick, was extraordinary. After one of them she told me she had had no energy – 'and that simply doesn't happen to me'. After another she was 'ridiculously tearful for a whole week, and I don't cry. Never have.' Another change was that 'I used to be able to drink a lot of alcohol without getting a hangover, but one day I got a brute of one after only two glasses of wine, and a few days later I had another hangover, and I was sick as well.' But the change in her periods amazed her the most. She didn't have the dull ache which always used to accompany it, the blood was brown rather than red and the bleeding was much less copious and only lasted two days.

'What does it all mean?' she asked.

'It's change, that's for sure,' I started, 'and basically change is good, for something has to change in order to stop all these miscarriages. I can't pretend to know exactly what's going on but I think it's change for the better. You are low on energy really – you've fuelled yourself on willpower. And grieving for what has happened seems to me absolutely appropriate, so I'm not surprised you cried, especially if you didn't at the time. And having a hangover is normal for most people. Your period sounds a bit more normal too. Perhaps your body used to suffer in silence but now that it is starting to work better it complains when you push it the way you always did.'

Anna accepted that. Indeed she accepted that getting better wasn't going to be a smooth process for her. Change was going to produce unpredictable effects; she was fine with that and it was a relief for me to hear it. It meant she wouldn't give up if things got a bit rocky and it meant that I could push things along without worrying that I was asking too much of her.

Just as well that we agreed on that because after two of her new-style periods the third was back to how it had been, but with the added extra of terrible pre-menstrual tension – for the first time ever.

'To tell you the truth, I always thought women who complained about it were exaggerating,' she said. 'Not anymore. I had tantrums over nothing; I picked fights with my husband when there was nothing to fight about; and the weirdest thing was that while I was doing it I knew it was ridiculous. I was sort of watching myself flying off the handle, seeing that it was completely over the top – but I couldn't stop. I was mortified by my behaviour, but I kept on all the same.'

Her next period was three days late. As she had always been regular to the hour, never mind the day, of course she thought she was pregnant, so when she started to bleed she crashed emotionally.

My first reaction was relief. I feared that if she got pregnant so soon and while all these changes were coursing through her body she might lose the baby again. I wanted more time for things to settle down. But it had brought her low. I pointed out that we knew she could get pregnant – that wasn't the problem – so she didn't have to fear that she couldn't do it again. She agreed. She said that she trusted it was work in progress and good progress at that, but when she spoke it was a bit polite, a bit formulaic, a bit like I imagined she must be at work. And that made me realise something I should have appreciated long before, which was the gap between the very organised and controlled front which she presented to the world and the rather tumultuous life that went on inside.

In fact, I reflected, I hadn't really appreciated the impact that bulimia must have had on her energy. The energy of the stomach goes downwards and serves to pass the churned-up food along to the small intestine. So when she made herself sick after a meal she must have been over-riding the movement of that energy and forcing it to do exactly the opposite of what was natural. What effect would that have, long term? I didn't know, but I could imagine that it would have undermined her system and left it chronically vulnerable and, if you can allow such a phrase, chronically confused too, as if it had constantly to ask – Do I do what I instinctively know is right or do I do what I am told? Do I keep this food in my stomach and deal with it as I feel I ought or do I respond to the pressure to release it in the wrong direction? Do I even try to do my job or just give up on it?

I was aghast that I hadn't realised all this sooner. If it was right then there were two enormous implications. One was that treatment should simply be directed to affirming and strengthening the natural movements of energy in her body; the other implication was that probably nothing I did was going to work if she continued to over-ride those movements. Changing her eating habits was going to be crucial. Binging and snacking had to go, and they had to be replaced by two proper meals a day, one of them hot.

Up to now I had been entirely upfront with Anna and told her what I was thinking and why. It's the way I usually work, and in any case I had instinctively matched the way she presented herself to me. We had got along fine on that basis, but I wasn't sure it would work now. Her bulimia, even though it was now much less of a habit than it had been, must have been a very deep-seated response to something which had affected her powerfully. No doubt it was the best she could do at the time and maybe it was the only way she could cope with whatever troubled or oppressed her. I didn't want to confront all that head on as I suspected it would be plenty strong enough to withstand a direct attack. Nor did I like the idea of turning her willpower against itself. Instead, I thought that it needed to yield and soften, to start to allow rather than to force; and surely that would be more difficult if I asked it to make the monumental effort of reversing a twenty-year-old habit?

So I decided that the best way to carry on with treatment was not to try to be too clever or too specific but simply to balance her energy as best I could. Then her body might start to send her clear messages to do what was good for her and stop doing what was not, and she might be able to hear them. This gave a new focus and direction to my work, and in my experience this always amplifies the power of treatment. For one thing treatments become clearer and more consistent, and that makes it easier for the body to respond and move towards health. It also makes me more confident of the points I choose, the combination of points I use, and the way I needle them.

So I was mightily relieved at her seventh treatment when she told me that she was eating breakfast and then two good meals a day. 'I haven't had a single sugar attack for three weeks. No sore belly either. I'm enjoying the balance of it.'

I was delighted by the word 'balance'. For the fundamental premise of all energy medicines is that health depends on balance. When Anna said she was 'enjoying the balance of it' she wasn't making an academic point, she was simply reporting her sensations and emotions so I could be sure that there had been a significant change in her energy, and that it felt good to her. It looked as if the new focus of my treatments was working. What I didn't know, of course, was whether or not this would stop her having miscarriages. And that raises a key difference between Western medicine and acupuncture.

If Anna's consultant had been able to identify a cause of her miscarriages then he or she would have treated it with confidence. Still, it might not have been the cause after all; or there might have been multiple causes and treating one of them would have been inadequate; or the treatment might not have been strong enough; or the patient might have reacted badly to the medication, or there might have been a strong psychological component which was untouched by the medication; and so on. There are countless ways in which the theory may not translate into a successful outcome. Being highly specific has its limitations.

Acupuncturists' diagnoses sound as if they are highly specific but fundamentally they are all diagnoses of imbalances of energy, and all treatment is directed to restoring balance. And just as with Western medicine there are countless ways in which this may fail to work for a particular patient – being highly general has its limitations too.

So with each new patient I ask myself – Is this person basically well enough that a Western medical intervention on its own would work? If so, perhaps I'll simply recommend a visit to the doctor. It may seem an odd way round – that you have to be well in order to use Western medicine – but there is a truth in it. Of course, it doesn't apply to life-threatening illness or disease, but I have often found that what looks like a sensible procedure according to Western medicine fails when the patient is fundamentally unwell. The patient just doesn't have the energy and other resources to cope with the intervention, and so cannot make use of it. I suspected that even if her consultant had found out why Anna was miscarrying, and treated her accordingly, it might not have worked.

Then followed a few months when she came for treatment looking well and continuing with all her new good habits.

Then she added a new one – she gave up alcohol, 'at least for the time being'. All good signs, and her energy was certainly better balanced. But there was something about her which gave me cause for concern. I couldn't quite put my finger on it, but when she turned up for treatment it was rather as if it was something she had valued in the past but was now more a matter of going through the motions. The sense of excitement and expectation of our early sessions had gone and had been replaced by a certain weariness. It was as if she had run an Olympic marathon and realised, a mile from the finish line, that she could only come in fourth; as if, desperately wanting a medal, it had all been for nothing.

However much a patient might want to be free of a long-term condition, the fact is that he or she will have got used to it and the prospect of change can be daunting, and I can't think of a more fundamental change than having a child. And I could also imagine her thinking, 'If I am so much better and I still can't have a child, then there really is something wrong with me; something which no one has ever found out, and now never will, as it'll be too late.' A depressing thought.

No system of medicine can take away the pain of these things, but one of the wonderful things about acupuncture is that it does recognise that being low in spirit is a genuine diagnosis and there are treatments for it. So now my job was to support her spirit so she could get to the finishing line and get there feeling good about what she had done. Of course I wanted her to have the medal, but I couldn't make it happen, and indeed the more I believed that it was the only goal the less I would be able to help her accept the outcome, whatever it was.

It is a fine line to tread. As a practitioner you have to care, but if you only care about one result, and if you think that it is entirely up to you whether or not it is achieved, then you are setting yourself up for a lifetime of stress and disappointment, and you are pushing your patients into an unhealthy dependence on you. For we are not masters of our own, or anyone else's, fate, and only rarely do we really know why things happen the way they do. My job was to help Anna get as well as she could possibly be, in body, mind and spirit as the conventional language has it, and then accept whatever happens. That acceptance is sometimes the hardest thing I have to do as a practitioner.

8

Ken's Chronic Fatigue and the Meaning of Health

THE CAR DIDN'T FIT THE VOICE. ON THE PHONE, when he made the appointment, Ken sounded like a slow, careful man, and there was a trace of apology when he spoke as if to tell me that he knew he was intruding on my valuable time and was sorry for it. Silly of me to base anything on this, but I was a bit taken aback when he arrived in an immaculate red Jaguar coupe. I couldn't help wondering if he had borrowed it. And indeed, as he locked it and walked over towards where I was standing to greet him, he looked back at the car with a trace of surprise and said, 'I've just bought it. From an old friend who knows about cars.'

'Very smart,' I said.

'Yes. I expect I'll get used to it.' He looked doubtful about that, and then greeted me with a handshake that was almost weak and a smile that was almost shy.

And there was something of the same contrast when he told me about his work. At first I got the impression that he was in some kind of routine job, perhaps in an accounts department of a big company. He told me, for example, that he was 'a cog in a large machine', that he 'pushed paper about' and that he 'had to go to endless meetings', so it took some persistence on my part to get him to admit that he was the deputy director of a very big national charity, a position of considerable power and responsibility. I wondered if his diffidence was an act that he put on to conceal a steely ambition and determination; if under its cover he had risen through the organisation without anybody quite noticing or finding any reason to object. Another quick judgement; but I did make a mental note that there might be two sides to Ken and that I needed to pay attention to which one I was going to treat.

He told me that he had had shingles twice. The first time was over a year ago. He had taken the anti-viral medication immediately and after ten days off work he felt fine again. The second time was nine months later, and although he had taken the same drug, this time he had now been off work for nearly five weeks. 'I was really unwell and Pat, my wife, got bossy for once – You're not right. You're not recovering. Go and see someone.' He smiled at the memory. 'So that's why I'm here.'

Mentally, I filed away the fact that it needed his wife to point out what was going on with him, and simply asked, 'Were you under stress, that first time?'

'That's a mild way of putting it. We had consultants in, which I didn't think was a good idea, but there was pressure to make savings and no one was quite willing to undertake the task. Anyway, the consultants ended up recommending a huge re-organisation which meant that some people would lose their jobs and others would be downgraded. I argued against it. The whole thing cut right across my principles and indeed the values the organisation stands for, but I lost. Then I had to implement the damn thing.'

'It sounds terrible,' I said. 'And this time?'

'This time I had to apply for my own job against outside candidates. I was really upset at the way it was handled, especially when the chairman had the gall to tell me that I needed to "embrace the process" – horrible phrase, horrible man. I spent quite a few weeks wondering how I'd hold my head up again if I couldn't even get the job I was already doing. I did get it, but it left a nasty taste.'

'Did you think of leaving?'

'I did. But I've been there a long time and I really care about what we do. Also, I think that I can at least mitigate the worst effects of the changes forced upon us. If any of the outsiders had got the job they'd have set about forcing us down a different road and to hell with a hundred years of devotion to our charitable purposes.'

I decided to start by taking a proper medical history. That had some surprises too. For one thing he got seriously ill every ten years, pretty much to the month. Glandular fever at twenty, chicken pox at thirty, asthma at forty and now shingles at fifty. What could possibly account for that? And it was unusual for someone to develop asthma for the first time relatively late in life. I asked if he needed any medication and found that he was using a corticosteroid inhaler. 'Two puffs in the morning and two in the evening. It keeps the asthma at bay.' I forbore to ask how he knew it did; simply noted that this was bound to have had a hugely depleting effect on his kidneys and hence on his general resilience.

The shingles had been on his forehead, both times, and had left him with headaches for the first time in his life. 'What are they like?' I asked. 'Disconcerting,' he replied. 'They sort of pop and crackle, as if someone's blowing through a straw, and then, soon after, I get shooting pains behind one eye and then, after a few moments, the other.'

'Does it always start with the same eye?'

He thought for a moment. 'No, it could be either. Which side it starts on seems to be random.'

I'd never heard of a headache like that before and I didn't know what to make of it, so I decided to think about it later and meanwhile check his pulses. They were weak and sinking, a bit better on the right than the left, pretty much what you'd expect from someone who was very depleted. I thought they might be a bit fast because shingles is a hot condition and even after it had cleared up there could still be some heat in his system, but there was no sign of it.

Next, the tongue. When he put his out I had to be careful not to gasp. It was extraordinary. Very swollen and very pale, shiny, with an enormous jagged crack down the middle. And as if that wasn't enough to startle me, there were small transverse cracks too and it was dry in the middle but wet everywhere else.

Ken's tongue spoke of so many imbalances and disturbances in his energy that it was far too complicated for me to make an instant diagnosis. So the first treatment was very simple indeed; I just needled a few points which I hoped would boost his energy generally and I told him that feedback would be essential. With it I could refine my ideas of what would help and each treatment could then be more and more accurate. Without it I would never know whether or not I was on the right track. I told him that I was looking for the obvious, how he felt generally and his energy levels, but I was also interested in anything that struck him as unusual or surprising, for that would be an indication of change.

I saw Ken a week later and he said that there had indeed been an overall change. 'It sounds contradictory,' he said, 'but I have felt more energised and more tired at the same time. I take it that because I have more energy I can appreciate how tired I've become?'

I said that sounded right.

'And there was one surprising thing. I forgot to tell you that since the shingles I've often found myself struggling for words. It was like broadband buffering. I would start a sentence and then stop, fully aware of how I want to go on but unable to quite find the next word. It would only last a moment or two, but it was disconcerting at the time. Anyway, that didn't happen this week.'

It was music to my ears. One of the very best things I ever hear from a patient is that something which he or she hadn't thought to mention has got better. It means I can't have been treating the symptom because I didn't know about it, so the treatment must have had a systemic effect. It gave me confidence that treatment would work well for Ken, even though I had no diagnosis as yet and there was no doubt a long way to go. I told him there were no guarantees, of course, but I thought the prospects were good.

I never say this to a patient unless I am as sure as I can be that healing is under way, but if I feel confident I like to say so. Many of the people I see have been through awful times, have spent months or years in a succession of doctors' surgeries and hospitals, have tried all sorts of medication, and often doubt that they will ever truly recover. So it does no harm to hear from someone with expertise that the prognosis is good.

At his third treatment he reported more change. First he said that his mood had improved. 'On the way home from you I couldn't stop grinning and I've been more cheerful ever since.' Then he told me that he had gone back to work, 'very part time'. There he had faced some really challenging encounters and at the time he had felt a slight tingling and warmth in the place on his forehead where the shingles had been. He was used to that; what was unexpected was his response to those encounters. Whereas before he would have felt under pressure and would have inwardly withdrawn himself from the situation, making himself rigid and unavailable, now he was able to stay present and, in his phrase, 'to ride the wave'.

There was something about the way he said this that made me think that he wasn't just using a conventional image, so I asked him if he had ever been a surfer.

'Oh, yes. I loved it. I was a real beach bum when I was younger.' There was warmth and nostalgia in his voice. 'Three or four summers I did little else. Lived in an old camper van, did odd jobs to earn enough to eat, and was out on the water whenever there was anything worth riding. It was great.' He smiled at me. 'You think I am a successful administrator but actually I am a failed surfer.'

I smiled back. 'Were you good enough to turn professional?'

'Maybe. But there were very few pros in those days and you do get tired of living hand to mouth. And then you meet a wonderful woman who is sympathetic to it all but who makes it quite clear that living in a van is strictly for one summer only. And then you marry her.'

It was a light exchange but I found it immensely helpful. I realised I had Ken exactly the wrong way round. The diffidence I saw in him when we first met was the laid-back surfer. It was the side of him that he didn't often reveal, perhaps a side he had suppressed ever since he had started work. Perhaps it is true of all of us that when we ignore or deny a part of us then it weakens our resilience and ability to heal.

All went well for the next few treatments and he reported each time that he felt better, had more energy, and felt stronger. At work, he noticed that he simply didn't feel the pressure as he used to. 'I've learned from all this that I really mustn't take it all so hard. I'll do my best and then...' He shrugged. 'And I am starting to enjoy myself again. At the weekend I rode my bike up Kentmere, my favourite valley, an hour and a half, it was a gorgeous day, I couldn't resist it. I couldn't have done it a month ago. I was tired afterwards but I slept well that night and I was fine the next day.'

I then gave him a treatment which made him worse. It seems to happen quite often that when a patient has done well from the first few treatments I then do one which goes wrong. Do I get over-confident, or slightly careless? Perhaps, I sometimes tell myself, it's simply that in the early stages of treatment almost anything is helpful – people who are starving don't tell you they'd prefer white bread instead of brown. Similarly, a body with depleted or disturbed energy will be glad to have anything that will help, but after a while, when it has recovered more or less normal functioning and has more specific needs, then it may reject a treatment which does not meet those needs.

I always tell my patients that they may sometimes get a reaction to a treatment. That is, they might not feel right, or they might get odd symptoms or even an aggravation of the problems that brought them to acupuncture in the first place. I add that it is usually the body simply adjusting to the change that treatment has brought about, and as long as it sorts itself out within twenty-four hours there is nothing to worry about – on the contrary, it is a sign that change is under way. But if they still don't feel right then they should let me know, because if treatment has gone wrong for some reason then the sooner I can put it right the better. Patients don't often phone, but three days after his last treatment Ken rang me up saying he had been feeling very sad and 'boggy-eyed tired' since I saw him. It was such a clear contrast to his previous reactions that I was pretty sure the treatment must be the cause; and if I had been in any doubt it was confirmed as soon as I saw him again, for his pulses were much worse than before.

There are so many reasons why a treatment can go wrong – mistaken diagnosis; right diagnosis but the wrong selection of points; right diagnosis and points but needled with the wrong technique; all the above correct, but too many or too few points used – and that is a brief list. But although I looked carefully for evidence of each of them I couldn't see that I had gone wrong in any of these common ways. It had to be something else.

For the first time I saw strain in Ken's face and for the first time he looked despondent and defeated. A tall man, he normally walked slowly, but this evening he shuffled. And his pulses were quite different too. At the first session there was nothing to suggest deep distress or disharmony; now they had such an uneasy quality that I didn't care to leave my fingers on them for longer than I had to – they had that sort of fizz you get when you bang your elbow in the wrong spot.

Maybe the previous treatments had peeled away layers of coping mechanisms and he was now down at the level at which his illness had originally manifested, or perhaps I just hadn't spotted the depth and intensity of his energetic depletion; in either case it was clear that he needed a much more profound treatment than I had done before. 'That feels like a re-boot,' he said after the needles had been in for some minutes. I liked the analogy. I don't know the technical definition of a computer re-boot, but I think of it as what you do when things are in such a muddle that you don't really know what is causing what, so there is no point trying to tackle each problem separately. Better to clear it all out and start again.

And indeed Ken's next report was remarkable. He had felt 'really cheerful, even elated' after the treatment and had been for two longer bike rides with no ill effects. 'But the most interesting thing,' he went on, 'was that I wanted to go out in the evening. Pat couldn't believe it. She is used to having to go out to films and concerts and to see friends by herself because, after a day talking to people at work, I just want to be on my own. But suddenly I didn't. And I enjoyed socialising. What happened? Do you know why?'

I didn't, and told him so. But I did wonder if the change was not so much in his social life but rather in how he was at work. I said that it might be that he had energy to spare in the evening because he no longer found his work so exhausting.

'Ah, well, yes,' he said. 'There is a difference at work. I have a warning light now, like on the dashboard of a car, the one that tells you it needs oil or you're running out of petrol. If I find myself stroking the place on my forehead where I had the shingles – I do it completely unconsciously when I feel some sensation there, not pain like it used to be, just a sensation, then I know I am feeling stress. And there are a couple of things that do it. One is when I am tired and I decide to push on.'

'Push on?'

'That's when I start a piece of work which might take a few hours and then, instead of spreading it over two or three days, I keep at it until it's finished even if it means working late or putting myself under pressure by ignoring other things that need doing. Anyway, I noticed last Friday that once I had stroked my forehead I decided to stop what I was doing and leave it till the following week. Which was good.

'The other change is when I get into a conflict. Last week I thought we weren't being open enough about something that had gone badly wrong at one of our overseas offices, and I was trying to persuade the director to make a clean breast of things. He kept saying he was worried about the effect it would have on our funders if it came out. It'll be much worse, I said, if when it does come out it looks as if we've been covering it up all along. But he's always been a short-term person – scared, really. Anyway in the old days I'd have kept on at it, would have gone off and talked to the other deputies to see if we could go to him as a group, might have rung up the chairman. I might even have leaked it, so as to force his hand. But now, if I find I'm stroking my forehead, I let it go. I've said my piece. I did my best. I can't make everything right.

'I've always had a passionate loyalty to the charity. All well and good, but not at the cost of my health. I'm not willing to sacrifice myself anymore. And funnily enough, I've changed in other ways too. In general, in ordinary office life, I am much more relaxed and tolerant of others and accepting of whatever happens. It's all just much easier. And not only for me, I expect,' he added with a smile. 'So what's next?'

'Tell you next time,' I said – I needed to mull it all over. And I ended up with two ideas. One was that his body had found a really clever way of telling him when it was time to stop – that instinctive gesture of stroking his forehead – and it was good that he was willing to listen to it. My other thought was to suspect that his newfound calm was bound to be tested; then we'd know how secure it was and if he was ready for the next stage of healing.

It was only a week or two later that an article he had written about the future of charitable work was published in a national newspaper. And, without telling him, they had cut the three crucial paragraphs in the middle of the piece, leaving it, in his words, 'Utter gobbledygook.' I held my breath. How had he responded?

'I was absolutely furious.'

'And?'

'I enjoyed it – in a perverse sort of a way.'

'Really?'

'Yes. The intensity of the emotion.'

'That's good?'

'It is. Hard to explain. Experiencing it without having to do anything about it – I quite liked that. In the old days I'd have rushed off to take some kind of action, and that meant I wouldn't have felt the emotion. It would just be doing the next urgent job on the list.'

I couldn't wait any longer to ask. 'And the forehead?'

'Oh, yes.' It was almost as if he had forgotten. 'I did feel the place but not for long.'

So it was indeed time for the next stage. I started to talk about his asthma and the effects of taking steroids for a long period of time. As a result, he cut his dosage from four puffs a day to two.

'How is it?'

'I've not noticed any difference. Do you think I am asthmatic?'

'Not really, no. I suppose you might have been once. But I've treated a lot of people with asthma and I don't see any of the signs and symptoms in you.'

'That's good. Oh, and by the way, I've gone back to work full time.'

'How is it?'

'Fine. Easy actually. So far I've left the office by five each day. If it's not done by then, whatever it is, it'll have to wait until tomorrow. And Pat has booked a holiday. I can't quite believe it. We're doing something adventurous again – kayaking off the west coast of Scotland.'

'Are you nervous about it?'

'Yes, but nervous excited, if you know what I mean.'

When he came back from Scotland he told me that he had given up the steroids altogether. 'It just seemed crazy, up there, in that wonderful air, to be putting chemicals into my lungs, so I stopped.'

'No ill effects?'

'On the contrary. It's a relief actually. And I'm learning to breathe again, properly. I never thought about it before, but while I was away, when I stopped taking the puffer, Pat told me that my breathing had changed. I used to take quick short breaths, like panting, high up, here.' He patted the very top of his chest. 'But I found I could drop my breath down so I was taking it from much lower, in my abdomen. And when I did I felt much calmer. I expect you know all about it but it was a revelation to me. Anyway I went and got a book on it and I now practise deliberately. It's made a big difference.'

'Wonderful,' I said. And when I'd taken his pulses I asked him to sit up so we could have a talk.

'When you first came for treatment you were in trouble, but that's no longer true. In fact, you are well and I am pretty sure it will continue. So we can either reckon the job is done and say goodbye, or you can come much less often and have treatment to maintain your health.'

'Oh, I'll come for maintenance,' he said immediately. 'No question.'

I was pleased but also intrigued.

'What makes you say that so quickly? I'm interested.'

Ken thought for a moment. 'Everything's changed and nothing's changed. I am in the same job, the same marriage, the same house, but it all feels different. I'm not paddling like crazy. When I was a surfer you could always tell the people who were really good because they seemed to catch the wave effortlessly. It wasn't effortless, but they knew which wave to leave alone and which one to go for, and when they went for it their timing was right so they were lifted at just the right moment and at just the right angle. It's a bit like that. I'm more skilful now. I don't have to keep trying to change things outside because I can deal with them more skilfully. I've learned a lot.'

'You certainly have.'

'And one of the things I've learned is health. I used to think it was the absence of anything wrong with me, but that's a ridiculous definition. Like saying most of the animals in the zoo aren't giraffes. It's not like that. I don't know how to define it but it's a positive thing. So I'll come for treatment to keep healthy and to get healthier.'

I agreed with all of that but I didn't add that I thought that one definition of health might be that there was no longer such a gap between the two sides of Ken; between, as he expressed it when we first met, the successful administrator and the beach bum and failed surfer. Perhaps illness follows when one side of us is denied and health comes when we find a way to bridge that gap.

9

Beatriz's Bad Hip and the Eleventh Session

BEATRIZ WAS AN UNUSUAL PATIENT. A TINY BRAZILIAN woman in her early sixties, a former professional samba dancer with six children, she arrived on a scooter and told me that she had no illness, no complaint; in fact there was nothing wrong with her at all. All of which was a first for me.

From an early age she had taken her dancing very seriously and had trained her body like an elite athlete. Then one day, when she was twenty-nine, she fell off the stage and hurt her back and left hip badly. It took almost a year before she could dance again, but she was never as good again. 'I have no pain now,' she told me, 'but the injury changed my life.'

To get well as quickly as possible she devised a way of massaging herself. The results were so good she started to show the younger dancers in the company how to do it too. The word spread, and more and more people turned up at her door asking her for treatment – first dancers, then actors and musicians, then sportsmen and women and then finally simply people with pain or disability. She had no qualifications but she was doing good work, relying mostly on what she had learned from paying the closest attention to her own body as she helped it to heal, but also using what she had learned from books and from feedback from her clients.

About five years before she came to me for treatment she had fallen in love with an Englishman, married him and left Sao Paulo for London. When I said I could hardly imagine what a culture shift that had been for her, she replied with a shrug, 'My children are grown with their own busy lives. My husband is English, he loves England and I love him. I am happy in a relationship – for the first time!'

When she first arrived she had no clients, so she decided she would use the time to learn more about anatomy, physiology and bodywork generally. She tried a number of therapies as a patient but was unimpressed – until she came across Structural Integration, more commonly known as Rolfing (after Ida Rolf, its founder). She knew immediately that it was the next step for her, so she signed on to qualify as a practitioner. Near the end of her training she read a book I had written and found ideas there that appealed to her, so she thought she would come and have one treatment from me as part of her professional development. That was ten years ago and I am still treating her, although less regularly nowadays.

In this last account I thought it would make a refreshing change to hear a patient's voice instead of mine, to have a patient's view of treatment instead of mine. So what follows is a conversation with Beatriz. Her English is good but not perfect and I have chosen not to change it.

I knew she had initially planned to come for one treatment only, so I started by asking why she had come back for more.

She shook her head. 'I nearly did not come again. It was so big that first time, maybe too big for me, I thought. So much happened. It was a lot. Let me see – how to explain?

'My life was hard. I could no longer dance, not as I used to be able to dance, not as I wanted to dance, so as well as the pain in my body there was a lot of mental pain, of sadness. And sadness too from my first two marriages, which were not good. Then I left my country, my work, my family to come here, and that was hard as well. But when I lay down' – she gestured towards my treatment couch in the corner of the room – 'with the needles in, all of it disappeared. I was lying there, feeling movements and changes in my body, coming, going, and that was all. Nothing else. Like, like…swimming.

'With swimming, you relax. The body floats. But you have to trust in order to float, yes? That is what happened on the couch. I trusted because you were taking care of me. You looked after me, you decided what to do, you took my pulse' – she touched her wrist with her fingertips – 'and you listened to me. Not to my words – to me. You put needles in, you took needles out. I could almost hear you thinking – what would be good for her – and I liked that.'

Beatriz nodded her head, agreeing with herself, as was her habit. I asked if she had noticed any changes later, in the days or weeks after her first treatment.

'What was amazing was my left hip, the place of the old injury.'

'You mean it was sore?'

'No! You don't understand. In that hip there is tightness, holding on, I know it so well. It does not move like the right hip, not as far each way, not as smooth. After that first treatment I did not check the movement of the hip. That was very unusual, very strange, because after other treatments, I always checked – it was so important, and I knew, to a millimetre, if there was a change. This time I didn't check; not once. You see?'

'Not really, no.'

'It just felt better. That was a new idea for me – feels better. I didn't know that. I know about pain and tightness and I know about more or less movement – but not better; just better, nothing more. Before, I always thought treatment was to fix something that is not working right. But this is treatment to feel better. And I know that my hip feels better, so why check? And then I, Beatriz, feel better too. And I think – is that because the hip is better, or does the hip feel better because I feel better? It is a good question, no?'

'It is a good question.' I paused. 'So that's why you came back?'

'Wait.' Beatriz held up her hand. 'It was not easy to come back. I was a little afraid. If you can do this, what else can you do with your needles? Will you find things I have to change and do not want to change? I felt some fear and some doubt of myself. That was new for me also. But it was good too, because after a little time I see that I can have fear and doubt and still be OK. That it is not a problem to have fear and doubt. In fact, that I have had them for a long time and it is better to see them. And anyway I know from the treatment that they do not have to stay. That is interesting. I do not have to think of them as part of me, Beatriz. They can come and they go like hot or cold, hungry or tired.

'All this from one treatment. So I wait until I feel strong before the next one! For sure. And it was different. I was different. This time I decided – I will see what he does. I will notice. I will try to understand.

'You tried to find a point on my leg, on the left' – she gestured to the place – 'and I felt the point when you touched it. But then you tried to find the same point on the right leg I did not feel it. That was interesting, because I thought that the left leg would be the one that did not feel. I decided I will ask you later. Why is this? Maybe because of the injury my left side is sensitive, or it needs more? Or what?

'Then the needles go in and I feel a difference again. A small pain in my left leg but no pain in the right. Then something happens in the right leg but nothing happens in the left. That one feels heavy; it is like thick mud. Two more needles go in. I wait. Now I feel a flow through my feet, like a tap turned on. Very nice.

Then one more needle, on the arm. Then nothing for a while. Then I feel a change in my heart.' Beatriz waved her right hand over the heart area as if she was wafting air through it. 'It gets more soft, more clear. That is very interesting to me. I did not know it was not soft, not clear, but now…I think maybe it was like a fist and now it is opening.' She made the identical gesture with her hand, fingers unfolding like a flower in the sun. 'I think, this is very good. No fear, no doubt, soft heart.

'Then nothing happens for a long time. You sit in your chair, I lie on your couch, and nothing happens. I think, he is a bit lazy maybe. He does not do much work when he works. Not like massage, not like Rolfing; they are hard work all the time. Then you get up and you do something with the needles, you move them or turn them. And then the same clear starts to happen in my head. That feels good too.

'You sit down again. I think – lazy again.' Beatriz smiled to show that she was teasing me. 'And I start to think, maybe this lazy is not so stupid. My body has time to use one thing before it is given another, and I have time to feel what happens.

'Then there is more change. The whole of the left of my body starts to get light. Not mud anymore. Then the two sides start to feel the same. I think – will they feel the same when I stand up, when I walk?

'And you take the needles out. I feel calm and clear. It feels very nice. So this is treatment to feel better. But still, I wait to see if it is only nice, like a hot bath, or if it does more.' She looked at me to see if I wanted her to go on. I nodded.

'One thing, it makes me change my work. After that treatment I take more time with my clients; I do not push so much to make the body go where I think it must go; I let it go where it wants to go. So it is good for my work. And good for me too – I am not so tired after working. But there is more.

'In my life I always made a lot of effort – to be a dancer, a top dancer, to get well after my fall, to learn to work with bodies and to have children – six children, is a lot of effort for sure. So now I stop and think, maybe I can be lazy like you. Maybe I can do what I need to do with not so much effort. So I try that. I think it will be easy, but no, it is not. First I make effort not to make effort! But then I learn not to try so hard and now I do more work with less work. I like that.

'Then, later, I had another idea. I thought – we are different, you and me. Your acupuncture works with the energy of the body; my Rolfing works with the structure of the body – bones, muscles, ligaments, tendons. Then I read in a book the words of one of Ida Rolf's students, a man she had treated many times in front of the class, to show them how to do it. He wrote about what it was like. He said that she was very strong and pushed deep into the body but she never hurt him – other people who did Rolfing hurt a lot, but she never hurt. He wanted to understand why. And he believed that she was using energy. In front of her fingers or her hand or her elbow, where she pushed into the body, she pushed energy first; and that energy opened the body so the fingers or hand or elbow could move into the space behind. Like the bow of a ship through the sea. And as I read his words I know I want to work like that too.

'So I thought, John knows about energy. Maybe I can learn from him how to do this. Then there was a surprise – you remember?' I nodded. 'You put two needles in here' – she pointed to her upper chest – 'then you sat behind my head and you put your hands on top of my shoulders and just left them there with a little pressure, very little, nothing more. And I thought – what is he doing now? And then came the first tear, out of the corner of my eye, one tear. Then more, then crying, crying, crying as if it would never stop. You did not move.

'There was no thinking about why I was sad or what had made me sad; there was just crying. So this crying was not from some idea, it was from the body. Inside the body was a lot of sadness, held in, and the needles and the hands and the crying together let it out. I felt much better afterwards. And Arthur, my husband, saw a change in me too, and it is true – I am happier now.

'And later I thought – my clients do not cry. Why do they not cry also? Maybe it is the needles or maybe it is something else. And one day, when I am working on a client, he starts to cry. And what a man to cry! A very tight man, stiff and tight and English. And I wonder – am I doing like the needles and your hands?

'Then I understood. With the stiff man – he hurt his Achilles tendon – I worked on his ankle, his leg, his buttock, but nothing happened. No change, no movement. So I stopped, I took my hands away, I waited, and then I put my hands back on his body, not where they were before but on the lower back, on the other side. I don't know why, I just trusted. And I worked there, deeply, and then he started to cry. And then I understood. Of course! This time I listened to his body and it tells me what to do for him. Now it is safe for me to work deeply and he feels safe too – so he can cry. Before, I listened to my brain telling me what to do to his Achilles tendon, but now my hands are talking to my client's body and my client's body talks to my hands, and we get along very good. No brain for me, no brain for him. No brainer!

'That is all. That is what I needed to know from you. But I still come to you for treatment sometimes. You know why? It is something from Ida Rolf herself. She said that a client needs ten sessions of Rolfing; after that the body is organised. But if a client comes for the eleventh session then treatment will never end. And it is the client's own fault. Because then the client has chosen to learn to be healthy – and there is no end to learning and no end to health.'

Reflections on Anna,
Ken and Beatriz

It is easy for doctors to see patients in terms of pathologies; to focus on pain, malfunction, illness and disability. But a lot of people turn up at their surgeries not with one clear-cut problem but with an array of symptoms which leave them feeling weary, stressed or unwell. Quite often they come with a vague sense of unease and say things like 'I'm not right in myself'. These patients do need help but Western medicine isn't well suited to address their complaints. That is partly because most doctors simply do not have enough time to really get to the bottom of what ails them, and partly because drugs and surgery – which are the only treatments they can offer – may well be inappropriate remedies.

Acupuncturists are in the very fortunate position of having theories and forms of treatment which apply to people who have not broken any bones, who do not have a recognised disease, and who are not suffering with the kind of temporary illness which, after a few days in bed, will pass without leaving any lasting trace – but who, as Ken's wife said so succinctly, are not right.

Perhaps the most fundamental thing these theories have to offer is a notion of health. With these people it is no good trying to identify an illness or disease because they don't have one.

But it is really helpful to try and identify what the patient would be like when wholly well, because then treatments can be devised to move towards it. This applied most obviously to Ken. He was suffering from the after-effects of shingles, but what really put him on the path back to health was the acknowledgement of the needs of his neglected surfer. And for Beatriz, a big step in her life and work was learning that more effort did not lead to better health, quite the contrary. It was true of Anna too, for although she had a clear medical problem, it was thinking about what could be right for her rather than what had gone wrong that offered a way forward.

So where Western medicine fights disease, acupuncture supports health. It is an over-simplification, of course, but it does shine a light on something which is often overlooked or misunderstood.

For acupuncture treatment is very different from Western medicine. There is no attempt to remove something wrong, like a tumour, nor to defeat a germ or a virus, nor even to manipulate a faulty body chemistry. In fact, there is no idea or implication that the practitioner will put something, anything, right. Instead, the treatment is designed to revive, to encourage and to amplify the body's own innate ability to heal – the ability which deals with a thousand difficulties and disturbances in each of us without our even being aware of it, and which has enabled the human race to grow in such extraordinary numbers over the millennia.

For Anna, Ken and Beatriz, their treatments brought about fundamental changes which, in the West, we would say was a matter of the mind rather than the body. Briefly, Anna did not realise that her diet and punishing exercise regime might be implicated in her miscarriages; and, like most people, she assumed that sooner or later a doctor would find out the cause of her problem and fix it. Ken was passionate about the charity for which he worked and, without thinking anything of it, persisted in sacrificing himself to its needs. Unwittingly, he had abandoned that part of himself which brought him joy and satisfaction outside the office. And it had never occurred to Beatriz that feeling better was a worthwhile goal, so when she could accept it she could also admit to her sadness, and let it go with tears.

Instead of thinking about these changes as a matter of mind rather than body, it is more helpful, I think, to see them as energetic. Much of our time is spent in habitual patterns of thought and in following mental paths carved out by long use, so it takes quite a lot of energy to jump out of these ruts and take new routes which can lead to new views and new destinations. Acupuncture treatments can supply the energy to do just that.

Is it simply the needles that supply that energy, or is there more to it than that? Most practitioners believe that the quality of the relationship with a patient makes a big difference too, but there is a specific aspect of this which can be overlooked. With all three of my patients I think it was the shift in perspective which provided much of the energy needed in order to jump them out of their mental ruts. It is an experience we have all had – of suddenly realising that we have been looking at something through the wrong end of the telescope, of knowing that an assumption or opinion, long held, is simply wrong. It happens a lot in romantic fiction. Elizabeth Bennet, in *Pride and Prejudice*, hates Mr Darcy because he is rude, haughty and indifferent to others, but falls in love with him when she comes to see that he is in fact kind, generous and fair. Converts, as they say, are the most passionate of believers, and it is the energy of that shift which provides the passion.

This is what happened, I think, to all three of these patients as they suddenly started to think of health rather than illness. Ken put it very well when he said that he had come to see how ridiculous it was to think of health as the absence of symptoms. Anna took on responsibility for her own health and Beatriz came to realise that she had volunteered for that eleventh session which will never end.

And there was another aspect to this shift of perspective which was important for all three of them. I saw it first with Ken when I realised that for many years he had repressed that part of him that loved to live out of a camper van waiting for the waves and then, when conditions were right, spending all day riding them. It occurred to me that when we repress an important part of ourselves we may also be repressing our ability to heal. That seemed to be true for Anna as well. She was such a dynamic woman and so good at being in charge of an organisation that it must have been really difficult for her to spend all those years putting herself in the hands of doctors and waiting for them to come up with a solution. So once she undertook the task herself I think it liberated something in her, something which had seemed to be irrelevant throughout all those hospital appointments and tests. And Beatriz had been so focused, so driven, that she had repressed her sadness. Once she was able to feel it she could let it go and start to become well.

Many of the people who are unwell have lost touch with some part of themselves or with something they have always wanted to be or do. These things are as real as their teeth or their lungs and they cannot be forever ignored without undermining their health. Perhaps it is through the combination of the wisdom of the past, summed up in the theories of acupuncture, and the immediacy of the treatment itself that people can see what they have lost and discover what they need in order to be well.

Conclusion

Healing and Health

Most books about acupuncture set out the general principles and theories and then give short examples or case studies to show how those theories were applied when treating a particular patient. This book works the other way round. That is, it looks to see what can be learned from experiencing acupuncture as a patient and practitioner. Are there any general principles to be deduced from the accounts of what happened in the treatment room? Do these stories reveal anything which could be of use to other practitioners and to other patients as they undertake a journey together towards health? And instead of looking at an acupuncturist's work through the lens of the usual diagnostic categories, is there anything that becomes clear from studying instead the immediate, the vivid and the sometimes confusing experience of giving treatment over a period of time?

What follows is what I learned from working with the patients I have described, both while I was treating them and then again as I wrote their stories. I discovered something about health and healing which I hadn't appreciated or understood before, something which I hope will help others to make the most of their time together. What emerged for me, from the accounts in this book, was that when treatment was successful there were three things that my patients and I had managed to do – and they were always the same three things. Equally, when a patient didn't do well with treatment I noticed that we had failed to do at least one of them. So I have come to see these things as the key conditions for healing.

Attention

There is a revival of interest in the art of paying attention. It can be seen in the enormous growth, in the West, of the ancient practices of mindfulness and meditation, and in the modern form of therapy called focusing. This revival comes, I think, from an instinctive awareness that the kind of goal-orientated, results-fixated, intention-driven effort so common in modern life often over-rides human needs and produces all kinds of damaging unintended consequences. And medicine has its instances too.

I met this emphasis on intention when I was first taught acupuncture, some thirty years ago. At the first session with a new patient my teacher would write down the next four or five treatments I should do. This casts the practitioner in the role of the expert who knows exactly what the patient needs and how he or she will respond to treatment, and it casts the patient in the role of the passive recipient of that expertise.

By contrast, a practitioner who works with attention rather than intention will come to each session with an air of open-minded curiosity. What is going on with this person today? What do I notice that is new? How has he or she changed since the last treatment and what does that tell me? Such an approach will naturally evoke a very different kind of response from the patient. While it may not be entirely conscious, he or she is bound to think something like – This practitioner is taking a real interest in me, not just in my symptoms but in me. He or she appears to want to know just why last week was so difficult for me, and actually seems to understand what it was like. Now, I wonder if there is anything else that might be relevant? – and so on. Instead of one being active and the other passive, they are both engaged in the process. This happened most noticeably with Anna, who quickly took on board that she needed to be a participant in her healing.

The same is true when needling. Instead of directing what is supposed to happen as the needle hits the point, the practitioner can see it as a suggestion or an invitation to the patient – 'How about this? Does it feel good? Can you make use of it, do you suppose?' The patient, again not usually consciously, will provide an answer to that question. Sometimes it comes through the needle itself – the practitioner might notice that it feels comfortable on the point; or it might feel awkward, as if it is trying to reach something it can't quite catch. Sometimes the answer comes from seeing the patient's reaction – is it a grimace or a smile that crosses his face? And sometimes it comes from taking the pulses straight afterwards. If the weak and deep pulses become stronger and fill out towards the surface, well and good; if they seem to shrink and sink then it's time to reconsider.

In short, it is through attention that patient and practitioner get to collaborate: each listening carefully to the other. As a result, the practitioner will be more inclined to ask questions which the rational mind would judge to be irrelevant, as I did when I followed up Ken's comment about 'riding a wave' and asked if he had ever been a surfer. And it makes it easier to notice those small impulses which may be wise; for example, not to needle the point you first thought of or to stop the treatment sooner than you expected.

When the patient pays close attention to his or her condition a wealth of information becomes available too. I once had a patient with chronic back pain which showed little sign of improvement after four treatments. It shifted around and varied in intensity from day to day. I could find no convincing diagnosis and was at a loss to know how best to treat it. At our fourth session I was about to say that I didn't think I could help when he produced fourteen sheets of paper – one for each day since we last met. On each sheet was the outline of a body and he had shaded with a pencil where he felt the pain at 6 pm, usually his worst time; the darker the shading the worse the pain. For the first time we could both see that there was indeed a clear pattern to his pain. That was the first breakthrough; the second came when he added to each sheet a few words about significant events each day.

This information enabled him to stop doing what made his pain worse and it helped me to treat him much more accurately than before. It took some time but he recovered completely, and it all came from his very bright idea of recording his pain and doing it religiously every day. Instead of it all being left to a doctor (first) then a physiotherapist (second) then an osteopath (third) then an acupuncturist (fourth), he was now involved in his own recovery. Instead of simply resenting his pain he became fascinated by it, and in return it started to give unmistakable signals as to what it needed in order to heal.

This is an instance of a much wider issue, one which explains much about why people seek help from acupuncture.

The flight-or-fight alarm reaction exists today for the same purpose evolution originally assigned to it: to enable us to survive. What has happened is that we have lost touch with the gut feelings designed to be our warning system. The body mounts a stress response, but the mind is unaware of the threat...

We no longer sense what is happening in our bodies and cannot therefore act in self-preserving ways. The physiology of stress eats away at our bodies not because it has outlived its usefulness but because we may no longer have the competence to recognize its signals. (Mate 2003, p.36)

One of the most important things that patients can get from treatment is a revival of their awareness of what is happening in their own bodies, and a sense of responsibility for their own health.

The second effect of co-operation between patient and practitioner is that it changes the energy of the encounter. Given that all acupuncturists rely on energy to help their patients, it would be ridiculous to overlook the importance of the energy that is generated between the two people in the treatment room. Naturally, all practitioners try to help their patients feel relaxed and comfortable, and to establish some kind of rapport with them, but I am thinking much more of finding a way in which the energy of each person can amplify that of the other.

The first time I observed Dr Fritz Smith at work, he was in his sixties. He did fourteen treatments that day and came out of the treatment room with a bounce in his step and a smile on his face. I was astonished and impressed. I was twenty years younger and I was exhausted after eight or nine treatments, the most I ever did in a day. What was going on? I don't know what he would say in answer to that question, but it seemed to me that both he and his patients were nourished and enlivened by the energy he initiated between them, and which they then generated together.

I noticed that it started right at the beginning of the session when he put himself and his patients on the same footing, simply as two people working together. So with one patient who had just qualified as an acupuncturist, he spoke for a few moments about the sense of a calling and the rewards of practice; there was no hint that he had many years' experience while the patient was a novice – they were both practitioners. With another, who was a doctor, he must have taken fifteen minutes examining her injured knee, talking all the time about the underlying anatomy and its typical distortions, before treating it.

And sooner or later in each treatment he invited patients to participate in some way. He might ask them to take a deep breath and feel how the chest moved; or to tell him what the sensation was like as the needle reached the point; or he might make a suggestion about something they might do afterwards to help the treatment settle down. All in all, it seemed to me that he was taking care to create an energy of collaboration in the room, one to which both of them could contribute and which would amplify what he could do by himself. I am sure it played a large part in the success of his treatments and I am sure too that it accounted for his own well-being at the end of a long day. As I watched him I thought – Who wouldn't want to work like that? And then – Who wouldn't want to be treated by someone like that?

Commitment

Going to an acupuncturist for the first time is a big step for many people. But sticking with treatment is an even bigger step. For one thing it costs money, and for another it means taking a substantial amount of time out during the day, what with travel and the appointment itself. And the chances are that it won't be clear for some time exactly how much it is all going to cost and how long it will have to go on for. Plenty of people must wonder if it is really worth their while, especially as results are rarely instant and unequivocal.

And even when treatment seems to be working well there are inevitably ups and downs. People don't get better at a precisely graduated rate, improving noticeably each week; in fact the rate of change may be quite bumpy. Even when a patient understands that what matters is an overall view – that the downs come less often and are less severe and the ups come more frequently and feel better – still, each time he or she feels bad again it is natural to wonder if it is worth persisting. And quite often there will be friends or family who insist on telling them it would be better to go to the doctor, or who suggest some other therapist who apparently had wonderful results with someone they know.

So it is no small matter when a patient makes a commitment to treatment and is willing to give it the time and attention it needs to work properly, and that makes a difference in and of itself. I often think of the time I was in a canoe on a big river and suddenly realised that there were big rapids ahead. The best thing to do in that situation, I was told, was not to try and head for the bank but to paddle straight ahead, right down the middle. I think that committing to treatment is a bit like that. It gives the best chance of getting through, and doing so quickly. In their various ways, quite a few of the patients described in this book did exactly that – William, Stacey, Anna and Ken, for example.

Commitment isn't always easy for the practitioner either. There are those patients who don't do as well as you hoped or expected and about whom you have worried and fretted – Is my diagnosis wrong or does it just need more time? What am I missing? Is it that she doesn't feel able to tell me what I need to know – and why is that? The list is endless and it is sometimes tempting to give up and recommend another practitioner or another therapy. Then there are the patients whom you find difficult. Perhaps they always turn up late, making you rush the appointment; or when, desperate for feedback from your most recent diagnosis, you ask them how they have been since the last treatment, they reply, vaguely, that they think it's all been more or less the same; or they agree to come weekly for four weeks but then don't make the next appointment until six weeks later – and then they turn up as if you can just carry on where you left off. Also there are those, of course, who resolutely refuse to take your advice and persist in doing things that are bound to undermine your best efforts.

But it is commitment to patients like these that often makes the difference. It may be precisely because they behave in this kind of way that they are ill in the first place. They do what they do out of habit, maybe because of some long-forgotten childhood strategy which made sense at the time but no longer serves them, and they will not get well unless someone helps them to change. Certainly it will take time for treatment to start to have an effect on such deep-seated behaviours, and it will probably meet with some resistance on the way, but the effects of a shift in a person's energy can be profound. To take the simplest of examples, once a patient starts to get relief from a chronic condition he or she can no longer hold on to the belief that nothing will work and no one can help. A practitioner's commitment to such a patient says, in language more powerful than words, that such beliefs are not necessarily true – and it is an essential part of treatment. I think this applied to Hugh, for example.

More effective than either of these commitments alone is when they are shared. Most patients try acupuncture because they are stuck in some way, stuck with an ailment or condition that isn't getting better, so it is possible to frame the whole of treatment as an attempt to help them get unstuck. Acupuncture, in essence, helps to do that by changing the state of the patient's energy but it is easy to overlook the fact that a shared commitment is an enormous source of energy in itself; and it may well be one which the patient has not experienced before.

On an average day perhaps as many as a third of people who go to see their general practitioner have symptoms that are deemed medically unexplained...amongst those with unequivocal, but undiagnosed, physical symptoms is a large group in whom no disease is found because there is no disease to find. In those people the medically unexplained symptoms are present, wholly or in part, for psychological or behavioural reasons. (O'Sullivan 2015, pp.6–7)

I have had patients like these who have been told, after extensive tests, that there is nothing wrong with them. Of course, that is simply sloppy language, because there is something wrong with them and they know it – it is just that 'there is no disease to find'.

If a patient realises that I am not going to give up, that I have been thinking about his treatments between sessions, that I have been willing to give him an emergency appointment at the end of a long day, and that I am willing to write a long and detailed explanation of what I am doing and why so that he can show it to his wife, it makes him more determined to play his part and do whatever he can to help the process along. And it works the other way round too. If I see that he has made the effort to go for a short walk every day and to resist eating a whole packet of biscuits with his afternoon cup of tea, that makes me more committed to doing whatever it takes to help him get better. We egg each other on, and that provides the most enormous boost to whatever the needles and the moxa can do alone.

Truth

I have had the privilege of watching three master practitioners at work and I have also spent quite a lot of time trying to understand what it was they were doing that was so special. One thing they all had in common, I noticed, was a profound acceptance of each patient and of his or her problems, however trivial, absurd, strange or heart-rending they appeared to be. That seemed to open the door to the possibility of transformation.

I think that acceptance has this effect because it encourages the patient to tell the truth about what has happened. None of us leads a blameless life, and when we have been foolish, when our spirits are low or when we have caused distress to others and to ourselves, illness often follows. Many patients sense this, if obscurely, so there is often some shame about the circumstances of an illness and its symptoms. Telling the truth is therapeutic in itself, especially if it has been long concealed, and it helps even more if that truth is heard with acceptance rather than rejection. And, of course, when the patient tells the truth then the practitioner has a much clearer idea of the source of the distress and what might be done to help healing.

There are many examples of this in the previous accounts, but the most obvious one is when Alice managed to tell me what had happened to her. For one thing it meant I could treat her more accurately thereafter; and for another it helped me to say, with complete conviction, that what had happened was not her fault. When I said 'You are not to blame,' she started to cry. Tears of sadness, but mixed with tears of relief too. From then on she gradually came to accept herself for who she really was, an innocent young woman free from that terrible self-judgement.

It seems that the clearer our perception of self approaches the truth, the deeper our capacity for self healing becomes. Where there is a very close correspondence between self image and truth, our self healing power may be virtually unlimited. (Upledger 1989, p.70)

There are a hundred reasons why our self image may be awry – pressures to be who our families required us to be when we were children; the unconscious adoption of strategies to get us through difficult situations; our instinctive response to the unexpected failures and disappointments in life, and so on. As a result we all have delusions about ourselves, we are all inconsistent and few of us live up to our ideals. It's all normal. And it's all a barrier to healing.

When I look back on my work with patients I can see how this issue has come up over and over again. There was a moment with Sean, for example, when he told me he had been bullied at school and used to hide in a place where he had to hang on with his arms. Then he added, 'I don't have to hang on anymore.' That was an acknowledgement of a truth and I think it was the start of his being able to leave the past behind. By contrast, Rachel, the brilliant mathematician who was out of work, could not face up to the reality of her situation – that she was never going to get her old job back and would have to find some new outlet for her enormous talent. She never did well with treatment and I think this is probably why.

Telling the truth goes both ways. The practitioner also needs to tell the truth, as best as he or she sees it. 'In the therapeutic process the single most important factor seems to be the ability of the therapist to reflect back the truth to the patient. Truth is the golden thread found in all effective therapeutic systems' (Upledger 1989, p.72). Plenty of patients ask us for reassurances we cannot give and invite us to agree with plans and proposals we do not think are wise. We do them no favours if we collude in a fantasy or encourage what we do not believe in.

> So the main responsibility of the therapist is to help the patient develop a truer, more correct self image… The art of therapy is sensing how rapidly the process can move without creating resistance or turning the patient away, and in allowing the patient to make his or her own discoveries. (Upledger 1989, p.70)

I think this explains why I succeeded with Sean and Alice and perhaps it accounts for my limited success with Pauline and her headaches. Her self image was so powerful that it never occurred to me to question it, nor to wonder if there was anything I could do to help her to 'develop a truer, more correct' one.

All this may seem more applicable to psychotherapy than the everyday practice of acupuncture, but one of the great strengths of this form of medicine is that working with energy affects the mind and body together. Patients may come to see themselves more clearly not through anything the practitioner says but simply because his or her energy is flowing as it should. Imagine a young man with low self esteem who gets a part in the school play and discovers that he is a very good actor; he will breathe deeper, walk taller, speak more clearly and have the confidence to go on and do well in other areas of his life. His success has changed his energetic state and that will have had physical, mental and emotional consequences. Indeed, it feels odd to even have to make the point; the separation between mind and body that we make in our culture may be how we think about ourselves, but it is not how we are.

There is one more overall point to make about what I have called the three key conditions of healing. I have discussed each of them separately but they aren't really separate. A patient who pays close attention to his or her symptoms and to how they change with each treatment is both learning about the truth and also making a commitment to getting better. Anna, who kept having miscarriages, did precisely this, and the results were wonderful (after an uncomplicated pregnancy she had a healthy baby girl). Similarly, a practitioner who is willing to tell a patient something he or she doesn't want to hear is both telling the truth and making a commitment – taking the risk, in the patient's best interests, that he or she will walk away. I made this kind of commitment to George, the violinist and craftsman; his back will never get better but I will go on treating him as long as he chooses to come.

And the reason why all these three overlap and end up amounting to the same thing is that they are all ways in which the patient and practitioner collaborate in healing. When they both do all these three things together it empowers the relationship between them, it amplifies the effects of their individual efforts and it adds a vital extra energy to the process.

Health

Most patients are used to the way Western doctors work, so they arrive at their first treatment with a set of assumptions and expectations which don't really apply to acupuncture and its practitioners. The procedure of Western medicine, in brief, starts from a set of known diseases and malfunctions of the body, sees which one has caused the patient's affliction, and then chooses a treatment to remove that cause. However effective this is for many patients, it is not always the route to health.

> …one of my patients…[was] a young mathematician with severe migraines. For him the resolution of a migraine, accompanied by a huge passage of pale urine, was always followed by a burst of original mathematical thinking. 'Curing' his migraines, we found, 'cured' his mathematical creativity, and he elected, given this strange economy of body and mind, to keep both. (Sacks 2017, p.154)

The phrase 'strange economy of body and mind' is evocative and suggestive. It speaks of the mysterious way in which the different parts of a person, which appear to have nothing to do with one another or may even seem contradictory, are in fact interdependent. So for each patient it may be necessary to have a unique notion of what will constitute his or her health.

In the following quotation a famous writer gives a startling example of just such a thing. He spent many years looking for a cure for his psoriasis – an inflammation of the skin that produces silvery white scales and itches dreadfully – until one day he found he was glad to give up the search.

> Only psoriasis could have taken a very average little boy, and furthermore a boy who loved the average, the daily, the safely hidden, and made him into a prolific, adaptable, ruthless-enough writer. What was my creativity, my relentless need to produce, but a parody of my skin's embarrassing overproduction? Was not my thick literary skin, which shrugged off rejection slips and patronising reviews by the sheaf, a superior version of my poor vulnerable own…? And with my changing epiderm came a certain transcendent optimism; like a snake I shed many skins… To my body…psoriasis is normal, and its suppression abnormal. Psoriasis is my health. (Updike 1990, pp.70–72)

These may seem to be extreme cases, but I think something of the sort is true of many of the people who come for acupuncture, and they present a challenge to their practitioners. For instead of planning treatment and measuring its success by the alleviation of symptoms, the acupuncturist has to try and grasp the whole of the patient's life and to discern what it is trying to manifest.

This does change the way both patient and practitioner view the process of treatment. They will agree that 'it's as important to find out what makes one better as it is to determine what makes one worse' (Yalom 1991, p.219), and will like the idea that 'A specialist in disease should begin his questions for diagnosis with issues of pleasure' (Moore 1992, p.164).

Health, in short, may not have much to do with the alleviation of symptoms but a great deal to do with the deep purposes and inclinations of a life. The impetus to health comes from the pattern, the interrelated organisation of a person's body, mind and spirit and its constant effort to renew, restore and preserve the whole. Acupuncture aids that effort. And in order to do so it cannot separate the weaknesses of the body from the disturbances of the mind, nor does it distinguish between either of these and distress of the spirit. For it appreciates that it works by harnessing every patient's innate ability to heal.

Writing about it in this way feels very clumsy because we don't really have words for it in modern Western culture. The nearest I can get is to say that we each have the capacity to allow our unique manifestation of life to be expressed to the full; and that acupuncture, at its best, provides crucial support to that noble endeavour.

Appendix
The Points

1. William's Irritable Bowel

I never arrived at a diagnosis of William's irritable bowel, at least not in conventional terms. At that first session the pulses suggested that there was a block between Spleen and Heart, which I treated with Sp 21 and Ht 1. I used even technique on the Spleen point and tonification without retention on the Heart point; which isn't what I was taught but makes sense – to me at any rate.

Thereafter, feeling that both the Large and Small Intestines were involved, I treated them directly with points like St 25, 37 and 39, Ren 4 and SI 4, 6 and 12. In addition there were a few treatments directed more to William's emotional state – Ht 7, Ren 14 and 15, and Bl 43 and 44. I suppose that a Five Element Acupuncturist, looking at this list, would assume I thought his constitutional factor was Fire. It may have been, but I am not good at that kind of diagnosis, so I didn't choose points on that basis. Nor did I choose points suggested by any particular syndrome, as none of the ones I know seemed to fit.

2. George's Bad Back

I mostly combined acupuncture with zero balancing – a kind of bodywork in which I am qualified. So a common treatment was to needle Du Mai – SI 3 left and Bl 62 right – with even technique, and then work with my hands while the needles were in. It felt a bit like having three hands – one working the channel while the other two attended to stress in the ribs and musculature. A similar idea was to needle Liv 3 with even technique so that Qi was being smoothed as I did the zero balancing.

I also tried Ah Shi points on the back, combined with either a distal point such as Bl 40 or 60, or a point on the Du channel such as 4 or 10, but I came to think that the distortion in his structure was too pronounced for these to give more than very temporary pain relief.

3. Stacey's Strange Symptoms

The first treatment was SJ 4, Pc 6 and Ren 15. Then I diagnosed what the authors of *Five Element Constitutional Acupuncture* call possession (Hicks, Hicks and Mole 2004, p.236) and inserted needles into the point just below Ren 15, then St 25, 32 and 41 bilaterally.

For the rest, my main impression of Stacey's energy was that it had been badly disturbed and so it needed to be calmed, contained and integrated. I needled Du 20 twice, both times with even technique; on one occasion combined with Liv 3 and another time with Ki 1. A similar approach but a different treatment was St 36, Sp 6 and Ren 12 together.

4. Sean's Hypochondria

Consistency and steadiness seemed to be essential for Sean's treatments, so I stuck almost exclusively to points on the hand and foot taiyin and hand and foot yangming. The first treatment was St 36, Sp 6 and Lu 9. I used these points often and at one time or another added Ren 8 with moxa, Ren 12, St 12 and 25, Sp 3, 10 and 21, and Lu 2 and 7.

5. Alice's and Hugh's Depression

With Alice I started with points to try and revive and lift her energy – Ki 1, Du 20, SJ 4, Pc 6, Bl 43. I then tried moxa on points on Alice's lower abdomen, principally on Ren 5 and St 26. After a while I used mainly spirit points such as Ki 24 and 26, Ren 17 and 19, and Ht 7.

My early impression of Hugh was that he was overwhelmed by grief, so I started with points like Lu 1 and 9, and Bl 13 and 42, done with even technique. I then tried moving his Metal energy by tonifying Bl 67 and Ki 7. I often paired points like these with Large Intestine points such as LI 4, 6, 7 and 11. In the end it was the upper kidney points that really helped – Ki 24, 25 and 26.

Two powerful books on the subject of the relationship between energy, emotion and illness are V. Hunt (1989) *Infinite Mind* and C. Pert (1997) *Molecules of Emotion.*

6. Pauline's Headaches

The first treatment was for Aggressive Energy (Hicks, Hicks and Mole 2004, p.229) – that is, Bl 13, 14, 15, 18, 20 and 23 – with the needles inserted very superficially. I next dispersed Phlegm with St 40 and Pc 5 and then moved blood with Pc 4 and Sp 10. After that I treated it as a Stomach headache, using, for example, St 41 and 45 with reducing technique; later I switched to thinking it might be a Liver one, so I tried Liv 3 with GB 34 and 41, also with reducing technique – which seemed to make things neither better nor worse.

Finally, what seemed to help most was to treat the severe headaches as caused by blood stagnation, so I used points like LI 4 and 11, Sp 6 and 10, SJ 5 and Pc 6.

7. Anna's Miscarriages

The first task seemed to be to warm her lower abdomen, so I treated St 29 and Ren 4 and 5, all with moxa – and indeed I continued to do this on occasion throughout the whole of her treatment. Next came the need to nourish blood and regulate the uterus through the Chong Mai, Sp 4 and Pc 6. I sometimes used Ren Mai, Lu 7 and Ki 6 for the same purpose, with the added benefit of supporting her Yin energy. Occasionally, I would simply nourish Blood with St 36 and Sp 6, or Bl 17, 19 and 20, and sometimes I treated the Spleen in order to help its task of holding an embryo, using Du 20, or Sp 3, 6 and 21, often combined with St 36 or 42 or Ren 12.

8. Ken's Chronic Fatigue

I started simply with St 36 and Sp 6. Then I switched to treating the kidneys, using Ki 3, 7, 10, 22 and 26 – not all at the same time – combined with points like Bl 23, 52 and 64, and Du 4.

The treatment that made him worse was when I persuaded myself that his constitutional factor was Wood and switched to Liver and Gall Bladder points. But interestingly, his reaction to these points seemed to reveal something that had been hidden from me before, which was the possibility that he was possessed (Hicks, Hicks and Mole 2004, p.236). I wasn't sure of the diagnosis as he didn't show any of the usual signs, but my instinct was to do the treatment anyway. Nor was there any dramatic response to the needles, though he did comment that he felt sadness coming up and, finally, when he was about to leave, he added, 'I felt a deep sense of calm lying there.' I was still unsure I had made the correct diagnosis until he returned for his next appointment when he told me that the treatment had brought 'great clarity and good humour'. Then he added, 'now everything seems possible'.

Thereafter I saw him about four or five times a year and he did well with very simple Fire treatments – SJ 4, Pc 7, SI 3, Ht 7, Ren 15 and Bl 14 and 43.

9. Beatriz's Bad Hip

In the first treatment I needled Liv 3 with SJ 4 and Pc 6, all bilaterally and with even technique. Later in the treatment I added GB 34 on the left only, to help the hip.

In the second treatment I cleared Phlegm with St 40 and Pc 5, and at the end I tonified St 36 and Lu 9 without retention.

In the third treatment I used Pc 6 again but this time paired it with Ki 25. Since then I have mainly used Fire points, though sometimes Kidney points worked well, and I once used moxa on Ren 8.

Much of what Beatriz reports echoes the wisdom and teachings of Dr Fritz Smith (1986) who was indeed one of Ida Rolf's pupils and on whom she often demonstrated her work.

References

Adams, P. (1999) *The Soul of Medicine*. London: Penguin Books.

Auden, W.H. (1976) 'In Memory of W.B. Yeats.' In *Collected Poems*. London: Faber and Faber (original work published 1947).

Eliot, G. (1994) *Middlemarch*. London: Penguin Books (original work published 1871–2).

Hicks, A., Hicks, J. and Mole, P. (2004) *Five Element Constitutional Acupuncture*. London: Churchill Livingstone.

Hunt, V.V. (1989) *Infinite Mind*. Malibu: Malibu Publishing Co.

Hunter, K.M. (1986) 'There was this one guy...' *Perspectives in Biology and Medicine 29*, 4.

MacPherson, H. (1997) 'Introduction.' In H. MacPherson and T.J. Kaptchuk (eds) *Acupuncture in Practice*. London: Churchill Livingstone.

Mate, G. (2003) *When the Body Says No*. Hoboken: John Wiley & Sons.

Moore, T. (1992) *Care of the Soul*. New York: HarperPerennial.

O'Sullivan, S. (2015) *It's All in Your Head*. London: Vintage.

Oschman, J. (2000) *Energy Medicine: The Scientific Basis*. London: Churchill Livingstone.

Pert, C. (1997) *Molecules of Emotion*. New York: Scribner.

Sacks, O. (2017) *The River of Consciousness*. London: Picador.

Siegel, B.S. (1990) *Peace, Love and Healing*. London: Rider.

Smith, F.F. (1986) *Inner Bridges – A Guide to Energy Movement and Body Structure.* Atlanta: Humanics.

Updike, J. (1990) *Self Consciousness.* London: Penguin Books.

Upledger, J.E. (1989) 'Self Discovery and Self Healing.' In R. Carlson and B. Shield (eds) *Healers on Healing.* Los Angeles: Jeremy P. Tarcher.

Weil, A. (2008) *Spontaneous Healing.* London: Sphere (original work published 1995).

Yalom, I.D. (1991) *Love's Executioner.* London: Penguin Books.

By the same author

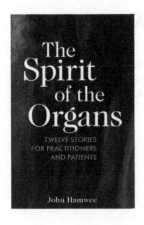

The Spirit of the Organs
Twelve stories for
practitioners and patients

Paperback: £12.99 / $18.95
ISBN: 978 1 84819 378 9
eISBN: 978 0 85701 334 7
208 pages

In the Chinese medicine tradition, understanding and resonating with the spirit of the organs leads to better diagnosis and more effective, powerful treatment. Behind most symptoms lies a disturbance of spirit, and the more alert a practitioner to the nature of such a disturbance the more effective the treatment is likely to be.

John Hamwee explores the spirit of each organ not in analytical, rational, summarising language but through life stories that express the nature and tendencies of the organ at a deep level. Through the stories of 12 people that embody the unique spirit of each organ, he shows the physical, emotional and spiritual nature of each, and their related tendencies and possibilities for improved wellbeing. Written to give Chinese medicine practitioners new ways to reflect on each organ in the most complete way, this book is also a lighthearted yet profound introduction to the heart of the Chinese medical tradition.

Intuitive Acupuncture

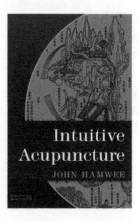

Paperback: £14.99 / $24.95
ISBN: 978 1 84819 273 7
eISBN: 978 0 85701 220 3
160 pages

The role of intuition is seldom identified in acupuncture training as one of the keys to effective practice. John Hamwee here explores its paramount importance in diagnosis and treatment, showing how development of the intuitive sense, and its appropriate use in the treatment room, is vital to building the most effective individual practice.

Through discussion of theory, clinical example, and the experiences of leading acupuncturists, the author shows how intuition, or the grasping of subliminal clues, can be developed, based on the practitioner's growing 'storeroom' of clinical experience and why it is so useful for this to become a conscious and rigorously examined process. He discusses the process of testing intuition against objective observation of the patient, and how an intuitive leap can provide a shortcut across an innumerable series of diagnostic steps, and lead to diagnostic and treatment decisions that make complete sense of the observable phenomena. He suggests that learning to trust the intuitive faculty, while still fully interrogating conclusions, is the basis of better patient outcomes and significantly advanced practice.

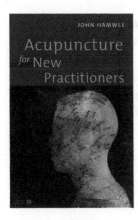

Acupuncture for New Practioners

Paperback: £12.99 / $19.95
ISBN: 978 1 84819 102 0
eISBN: 978 0 85701 083 4
160 pages

An invaluable guide for anyone beginning a career in acupuncture, this book offers a unique and supportive insight into the challenges and the pitfalls that the novice acupuncturist is likely to encounter, and provides encouragement and down-to-earth ideas for tackling them.

Written in an easy-to-read conversational style with useful case studies throughout, this book will help newly-qualified acupuncturists to reflect on what kind of practitioner they want to be. It addresses styles of working, common mistakes, confidence with patients, becoming a better practitioner, and how to think about success and failure in the treatment room. The ultimate goal is to ensure that the practitioner ends the day refreshed and enlivened by the work and has confidence in the treatments given.

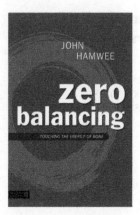

Zero Balancing
Touching the Energy of Bone

Paperback: £14.99 / $24.95
ISBN: 978 1 84819 234 8
eISBN: 978 0 85701 182 4
144 pages

The definitive guide to Zero Balancing brings this increasingly popular therapy to life. It contains a clear description of the anatomy and physiology of energy which leads on to a compelling explanation of how and why this form of bodywork can have such powerful effects. Throughout, there are illustrations which convey the unique energy of a Zero Balancing session and John Hamwee provides fascinating examples of clients, their experiences and the outcomes of the work.

Of related interest

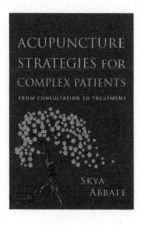

**Acupuncture Strategies
for Complex Patients**
**From Consultation
to Treatment**
Skya Abbate

Paperback: £25.00 / $35.00
ISBN: 978 1 84819 380 2
eISBN: 978 0 85701 336 1
264 pages

Written by an experienced acupuncturist and educator, this advanced textbook provides strategies which support the foundational energy of a person, including their qi, blood, yin, yang and essence. The book takes an integrative approach, providing insightful recommendations relating to diagnosis and the construction of treatment plans. It shows how needling strategies are connected to rules of point selection, the point classification system, and nourishing the foundational energies of patients. Techniques such as bloodletting, gua sha and the eight extraordinary meridians are covered, and the book is supported by clear illustrations, chapter summary charts and template patient handouts. Ideal for use as a practical manual for practitioners of acupuncture, it is also useful as a student textbook.

Skya Abbate has been a practising acupuncturist for over three decades, and is an experienced and senior teacher at Southwest Acupuncture College. She has published books on Auricular Acupuncture, Palpatory Diagnosis and Advanced Techniques in Oriental Medicine.